Welcome!

I hope you find this guide useful. These are things I have learned from my time performing. This book is designed to help you look at all angles of performing and build on your own experience. Providing tools to help you visualise and break down techniques, this book will help you develop your performance skills. Use this manual as much or as little as you need to focus your ideas and compartmentalise different aspects of performing. Make sure that you don't miss anything on the performance journey. Enjoy the show!

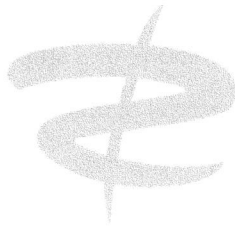

A quick thanks...

Thank you to all those who have been on this performing journey with me. It has been an amazing ride, and influenced by amazing artists. Thank you for being a part of it! Whether that be by guiding, performing, learning or teaching, you are all amazing inspirations, thank you! Jed, Mel, Mikku, Danni and my amazing family for helping me proof read my little project! My husband, for his amazing patience with my little projects I come up with. Also, a quick thankyou to Deric Martin for the cover photo and the photo in the book. And to Rejis Chibanda for the back cover image.

Now to get personal; as a special thanks to Granddad for introducing me to the theatre, our days at The Grand are memories I hold very dear. Mum for her community theatre days, and patience driving me around from one performing art to another growing up. And finally, my father; growing up in the back of the room with you up on stage presenting seems to have made an influence on my direction as I grew up!

Act Creation by Lara Johnson

Disclaimer

I am a pole fitness instructor and not a health professional. This workbook provides general information about pole fitness and burlesque. It does not consider your personal circumstances in any way. This workbook contains excerpts from *The First Steps* – Instructors Edition and *Personal Pole and Aerial Record*, both books written by Lara Johnson and published by Rapture Arts.

Pole fitness is a high-risk sport. Please consult a health professional before starting any fitness program to ensure that it is right for your needs and abilities. Do not start a pole fitness program if your instructor or healthcare provider advises against it. With all dance and fitness, please monitor and work within your own limitations, and stop immediately if you experience symptoms of faintness, dizziness, pain, or shortness of breath at any time while exercising. Remember that your body needs to rest. Training regimes need to allow for rest and recovery. In order to perform well, you must work within your limits and look after your body.

This guide is not a substitute for skilled instruction. The author recommends seeking professional support from a pole fitness or dance instructor before attempting a pole fitness or dance program on your own. This means that you will have a competent individual to assist you if needed. Please ensure that your pole or prop setup and area is secure and safe as per manufacturer specifications. Ensure an unobstructed space for both training and performing.

To the extent permitted by law, the author of this book disclaims any liability (including negligence) arising directly or indirectly from your use of the information contained in this workbook.

First Edition 2022

Act Creation by Lara Johnson

Table of Contents

Introduction

People often think that putting a show together is easy. For some people, it may be more natural. For others, there is a complex list of considerations and unknowns that can make performing an overwhelming and daunting experience. This manual is here to help by providing information on aspects of performing you may not have considered. This guide will help to break difficult concepts into manageable steps. You can use this manual to help you plan and create your own unique character and performance.

I have been onstage in a variety of performance styles since I was a child. I have learned from some of the greats and have been asked by many to help them put together their own shows. Here, I have provided much of my knowledge and experience to help you stand out and be uniquely you onstage. This book is designed to help you put together the performance you've been imagining and to help it not feel like the weight of the world is on your shoulders when you're working out.

The next page will give you a snapshot of what we're looking at in this manual. We will follow this outline through the steps of creating an act and look at a range of different ways of doing things along the way.

Act Creation in a Snapshot

Step 1: Brainstorming Ideas

Divide your ideas into themed groups, and break down the core of what inspires you. Doing a moves-specific brainstorm would be separate. This is more focused on theme, style, and character elements. Research the core theories, values, and stories behind your inspiration. Bring out an aspect that resonates with you to use as the inspiration for your show.

Step 2: Brainstorming Your Performance

Using the same brainstorming method, start to think about what you want to include in your performance. Consider themes, storylines, moves, transitions, lines, character changes, and costume changes. Don't forget about lights, voiceovers, and special effects!

Step 3: Breaking Down Characters

Use character breakdown sheets to start visualising your character and performing persona. Give your persona a name and an identity to help you understand who they are and how they perform onstage.

Step 4: Planning the Show

Now that you know who your character is, work on how your character moves and acts to start putting together your show. Don't set the bar too high during the creation stage. Don't set yourself too many restrictions. Allow the creative juices to flow and develop. Set a consistent training routine, and use that time to work on your performance. Your training routine can be as simple as a set amount of time, or a number of days per week. As long as you continue to progress, you're fine. You don't need to force it or put pressure on yourself. Once the choreography is set, you can section out areas to work on. Working on one small section with just a few moves repetitively can help you to really get to know the cleanest pathway and nicest line or angle. Not only does it help to get it in your brain but it really helps to clean up the movements to make the transitions crisp. You can then confidently move onto the next section, or "moment" to work on.

Step 5: Record Your Routine

Next, record what you're feeling and visualising so far so that you can neaten lines, remove fluff, and make movements purposeful. This is your chance to pull apart the elements you like and change the things you don't. Find things you want to do, and get these things sorted first. Then brainstorm and fill in the gaps, making everything mesh together. This way, you won't get lost by starting at the beginning; there is no need to start here and potentially get frustrated finding your flow. Start with the flow. Work on the parts that work easily for you before bringing in other elements and joining it together. Elements that are good to consider are variances in direction, speed and height, as well as the weight of the movement, is it heavy or light. Once you have a routine, it's time to practise, neaten, and finalise.

Step 6: Consider Staging

Staging is the next important consideration. You'll need to think about how to use your stage, marking out your movements and integrating opportunities for audience engagement. Your audience is there, acknowledge them. You might also need to consider lighting and costuming. Will you disappear in the space, or will your space allow you and your colours to stand out? Remember to make provisions for sound and special effects. Learn to read the room. Does your performance match the vibe and demographic of your target audience?

The room is filled with darkness except for one stream of light coming down like a ray of moonlight, illuminating a perfect circle on the wooden floor. The red velvet curtains hang heavy beside you, and the air is buzzing with excitement and anticipation. The stage feels like a great expanse, going on forever. But once you step into a mottled crowd of dark shadows, you realise it is only a few steps. It is time. You are here. The show will go on!

You are preparing for the moment before stepping out from behind the curtains—and, of course the moments that follow. How much planning goes into getting a show to this point? This is what you're here to do.

Welcome to the stage!

Act Creation by Lara Johnson

Brainstorm Your Inspiration

Let's start the journey. Your act starts with ideas. You want to work out what your ideas are. If you have more than one, you can decide how they relate to each other or what they have in common. It's time to start recording your inspiration.

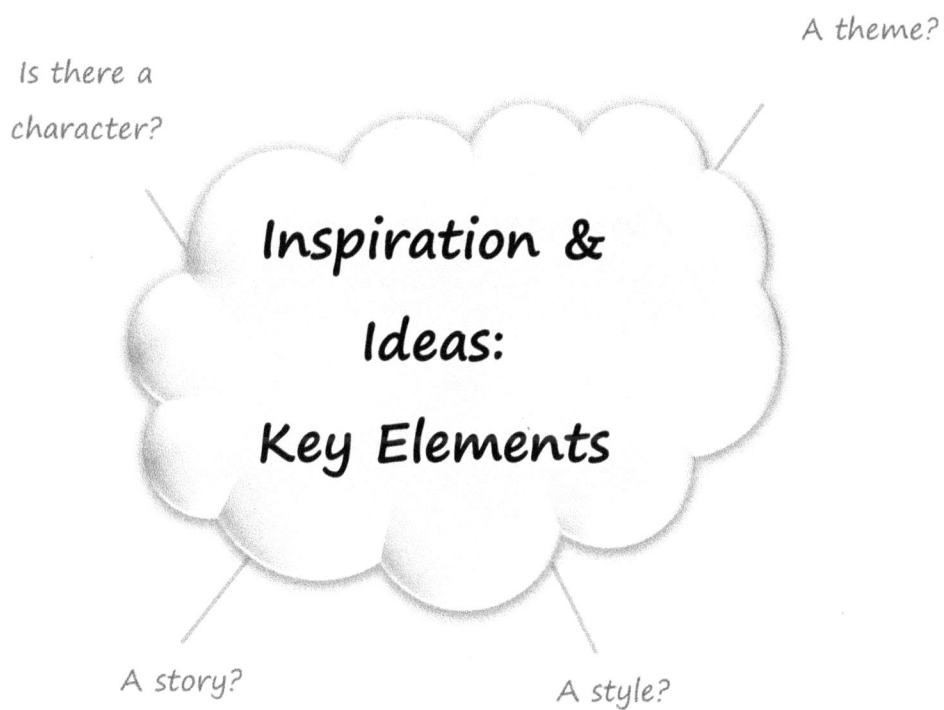

A theme?

Is there a character?

Inspiration & Ideas: Key Elements

A story?

A style?

Brainstorm Your Inspiration

In the first brainstorm, you identified your main ideas and inspiration. Use this second brainstorm to help you communicate your inspiration and ideas with the audience.

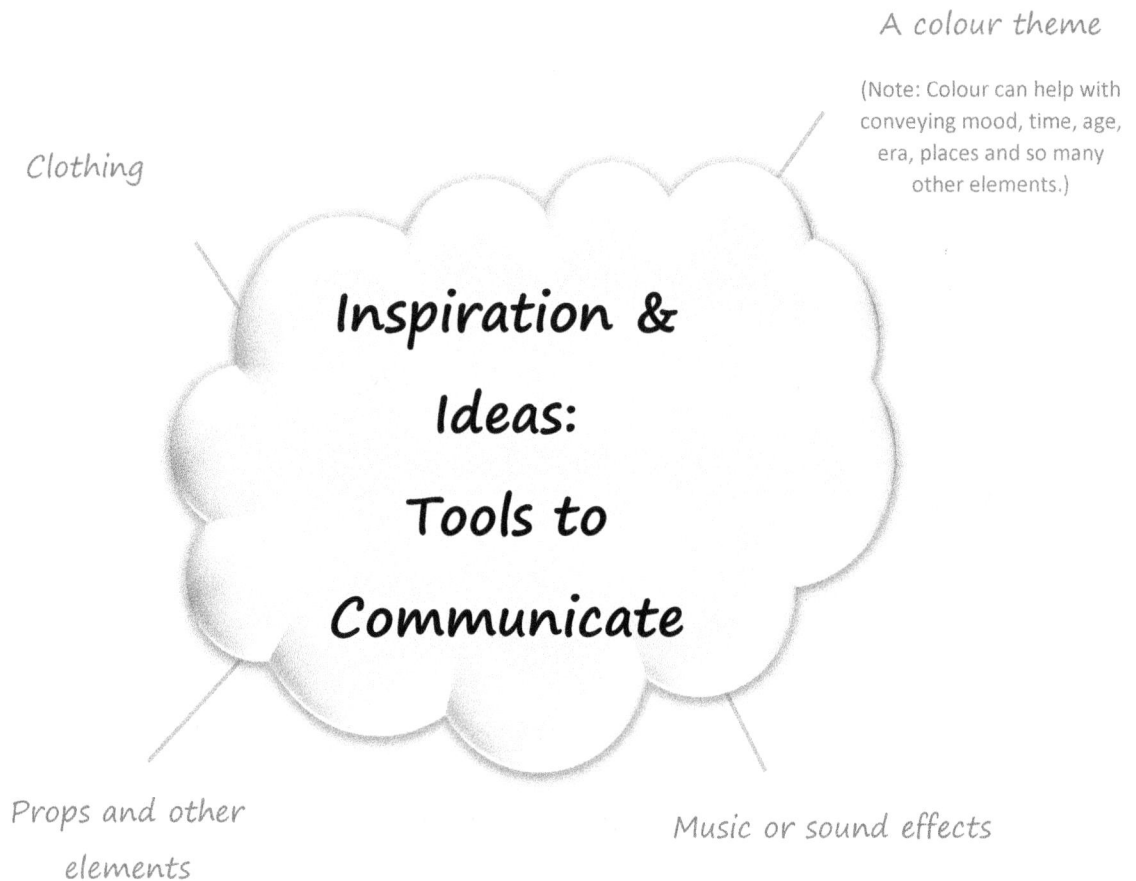

A colour theme

(Note: Colour can help with conveying mood, time, age, era, places and so many other elements.)

Clothing

Inspiration &
Ideas:
Tools to
Communicate

Props and other elements

Music or sound effects

These are considerations that will help you communicate your inspiration and ideas with the audience. Use your senses, and consider what the audience will see, feel, and hear. Use these elements to enhance your performance.

Examine Your Ideas

List your ideas to make brainstorming feel a little more manageable. See where your inspirations truly lie, and break down how you can create your perfect show by drawing from what inspires you. Can some of your ideas intertwine or combine? Is there a common theme?

Common Characters

_____

_____

_____

_____

_____

_____

Common Themes

_____

_____

_____

_____

_____

_____

Common Storylines or Genres (This may include mythologies, countries, anything.)

_____

_____

_____

_____

_____

Do Your Research

Are there any values, quotes, characters, or historical events that relate to your theme? What stands out to you in your research? List these things here, and come back to them when you're putting your routine together to see if they inspire you or relate to the show you're creating.

_____

_____

_____

_____

_____

_____

_____

_____

_____

_____

_____

_____

_____

Why are you doing all of this? Great communicators are storytellers! Your performance is a story, whether it is a literal story or a story of the heart. It has a meaning, and understanding the ins and outs of this helps you communicate your story with your audience. This helps to draw audiences in with your performance.

One thing to be aware of is that you don't want to use the same song, act, or concept as other acts. This is a tricky concern at times, as you never really know who is doing what. But you can research other shows and ensure that you are doing something different. With this said, I have done great shows at events where multiple acts used the same popular song. This is a huge thing in the burlesque community!

Brainstorm Your Routine

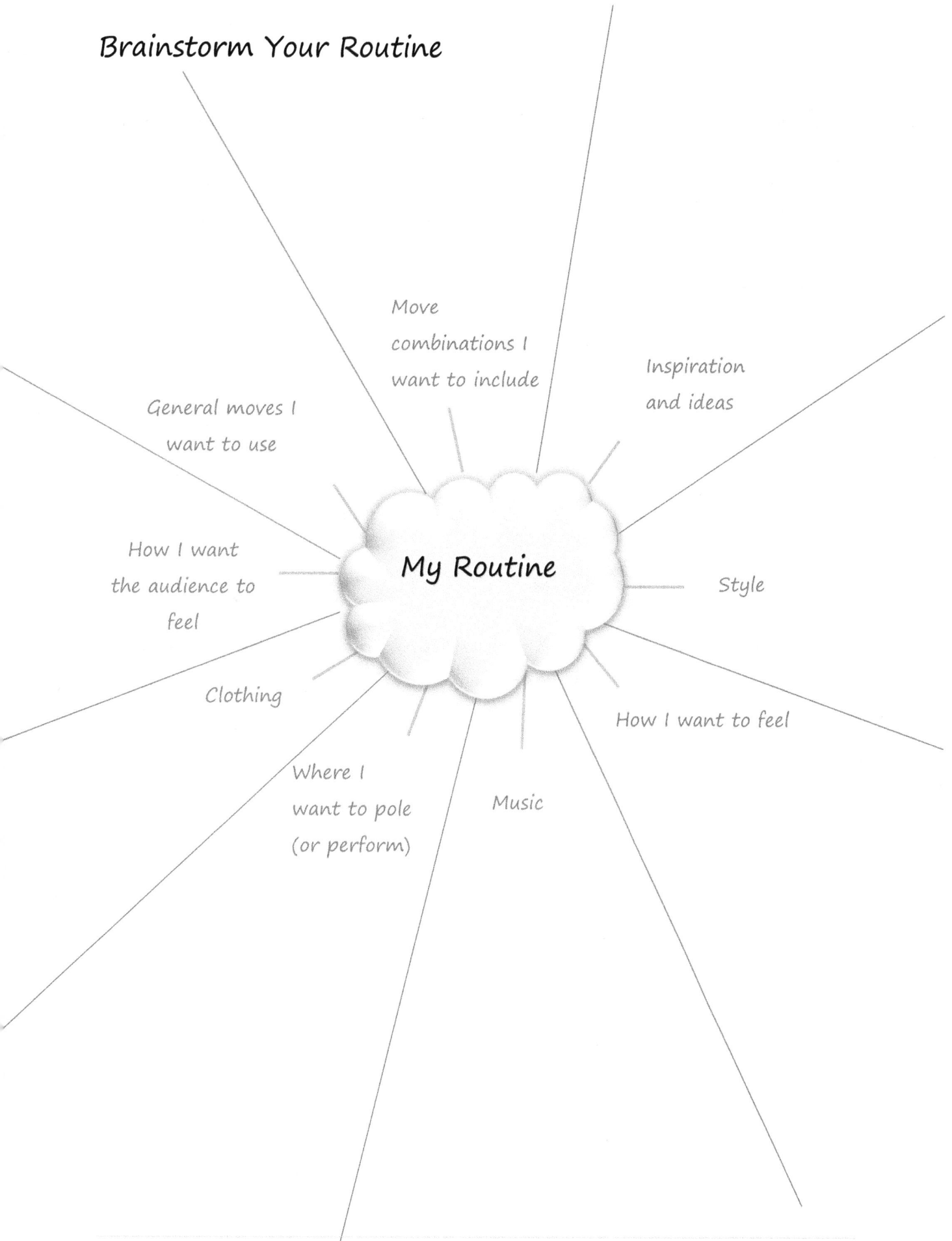

My Routine

Move combinations I want to include

Inspiration and ideas

General moves I want to use

How I want the audience to feel

Style

Clothing

How I want to feel

Where I want to pole (or perform)

Music

Visualisation

This is so important! Seeing is believing, and seeing the steps and the event helps you make it a reality.

How your Performance Looks
(This could be any product of your performing goal, if your goal is to boost confidence, how does that look as you walk down the street, or present yourself?)

_____

_____

_____

How It Makes Me Feel

_____

_____

_____

Steps I Need to Take to Achieve My Visual Goal

Working out what actions or steps you need to take is an important first step. Setting a date provides you with motivation and keeps you accountable to your goal. Feel free to use whatever motivation method works for you.

Steps	Achieved By	Completion Date

Vision Boards

In a snapshot, a vision board is a place to record all your dreams and desires for your act. How you do this is up to you.

Why create a vision board?

✓ It can help you visualise your goal. Seeing is believing!

✓ It can increase your motivation, focus, productivity, and determination.

✓ It increases your chance of success.

✓ It clarifies what you want and makes the dream real in your mind.

✓ It creates an emotional connection, which helps with motivation.

What is a vision board?

A vision board is unique to you. Many people use a collage of pictures, but it can also be a compilation of words, colours, styles, or other things you find that resonate with you. Basically, a vision board is a place for your dreams and desires. You can put your board in a place where you'll see it regularly so that it can motivate you to work towards your dreams. Visualisation is a strong tool in helping to make your dreams a reality. After all, if you haven't dreamed it, how do you know it's what you want to do? Your vision board is a constant reminder of what your goal looks like.

How to create a vision board

How you create your vision board is up to you. A visual person will search for images that inspire them and set a mood. Other people may go in with a mission for what they want to achieve. It's all about the final intention and taking the path that works for you.

- Think about your goals, and break them down.
  - What activities, styles, and moves do you want to learn?
  - Is there something you want to get better at? Straight lines, pointed toes, or deadlifting strength? What makes this move feel right to you?
  - What is the next step? Have you set a personal goal, a career goal, or a goal to achieve the perfect move for a photoshoot?
- Believe in your goals and yourself!
- What is your theme? Is it particular to a move or an event, or is it a style of movement?
- Decide whether you want a specific vision board or a more generalised one, reflecting a style, a flow, or even a look.

- Now start creating. Pick your style or format, and find images, sounds, colours, and words to add to it. Keep it positive, and get creative with scissors and glue. Another option here is to use Pinterest. The important thing is to get into your creative space! Do you need photos? Articles? Magazines? Little bits of nature? Quotes or lines from books? This is yours, use what resonates with you!

You will not feel creative every day or even every week. This is normal, so don't stress. Just flow with it. Recognise when you need to rest and when you are ready to create. Some days, things don't work creatively, but there are always other things that you can work on to continually progress.

My Vision Board

An extra space for any notes, pictures, website links. A space to write or draw or cut and paste whatever you need to add to your vision board!

You walk into a saloon bar. The air is hazy and filled with the smell of spilt drinks. A mystical voice drifts through the air. Having not quite gotten to the point of looking up, you notice the curves saunter towards you, one slow step at a time. The light bounces off the curves of their hips. You feel as if you're lost in a mesmerising moment in time. As your eyes travel up, every curve becomes apparent, and you sink down in your seat. Everything about this moment has made you stop and hold your breath. You have come face-to-face with Jessica Rabbit.

Iconic characters like Jessica Rabbit, or even Betty Boop, are stuck in time. They have a recognisable look and vibe about them. Think about how they move and act. They are so very *them*. What is your character going to be like?

Create Your Character

Now it's time to create your character. Knowing what your character looks like helps you work out how they move and dress. Remember to consider whether your costume will limit or promote certain moves. Think about how your gestures and movements work together to develop your onstage persona. This includes hand, feet and even head movements. Consider how your character can evolve throughout the show, allowing the audience to connect with the routine. Don't forget to name your character! This is a strangely important element.

Character Notes

_____

_____

_____

_____

_____

_____

Personality Traits

_____

_____

_____

_____

Mood or Style of Performance or Movement

_____

_____

_____

Signature Moves, Props, or Reactions

_____

_____

_____

_____

Play with your character and gestures. Look at high movements, low movements, fast movements, and slow movements. Look at how your character walks. If you have an apparatus, play with your character outside or off your apparatus in its own environment. Think about character-defining movements or patterns. Focus on different parts of your body, and feel how your character moves (yes, even focus on the unusual things, like shoulders!). Have some fun with it! Explore and play.

This helps you find the real character, letting go of inhibitions and playing in this zone. I've done this in the dark with the lights off. You can even do this blindfolded in a highly controlled, risk-managed environment. This helps to take out some of your senses so you can feel the movement more. Please be careful and manage risk appropriately with someone around to help you if needed. Developing your character in this way helps you decide who they will be in your routine.

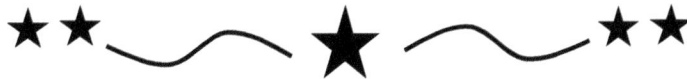

★ ★ ⌒ ★ ⌒ ★ ★

I also find understanding the song very important to developing your Character, your song is part of your image. We will revisit this in another section, but thinking about it early helps to put it all together.

Song Notes and Notable points

_____

_____

_____

Feelings that the song evokes in you

_____

_____

Meaning behind the song

_____

_____

_____

_____

_____

_____

Plan Your Character's Image

Decide on styles, colours, makeup looks, and more as you plan your character.

(makeup face maps are readily found online for those wanting an alternative format)

Eyes:

Eyebrows:

Eyeshadow:

      Base colour:

      Crease:

      Outer corner:

      Inner corner:

      Inspiration:

Eyeliner:

Lower lash line:

Mascara:

Lashes/lash style:

Contacts/glasses:

Outer eye features:

Gems or embellishments:

Hair:

Colour:

Style:

Products needed:

Feature:

Hat/headdress:

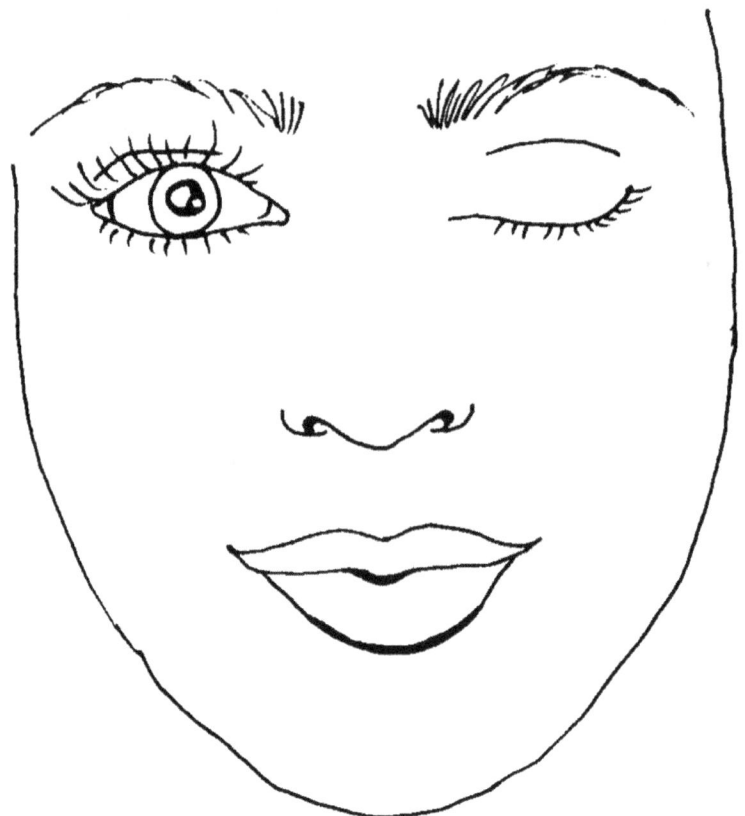

Face:

Primer:

Concealer:

Foundation:

Powder:

Blush:

Bronzer:

Contour:

Highlight:

Setting spray:

Accessories: (glitter? gems?)

Inspiration:

Lips:

Liner:

Gloss:

Colour:

Lipstick:

Embellishments or detail:

Lip Shape (era related):

Plan Your Character's Image

Decide on styles, colours, makeup looks, and more as you plan your character.

Eyes:

Eyebrows:

Eyeshadow:

     Base colour:

     Crease:

     Outer corner:

     Inner corner:

Eyeliner:

Lower lash line:

Mascara:

Lashes/lash style:

Contacts/glasses:

Highlights or embellishments:

Inspiration:

Hair:

Colour:

Style:

Feature:

Hat/headdress:

Product Needed:

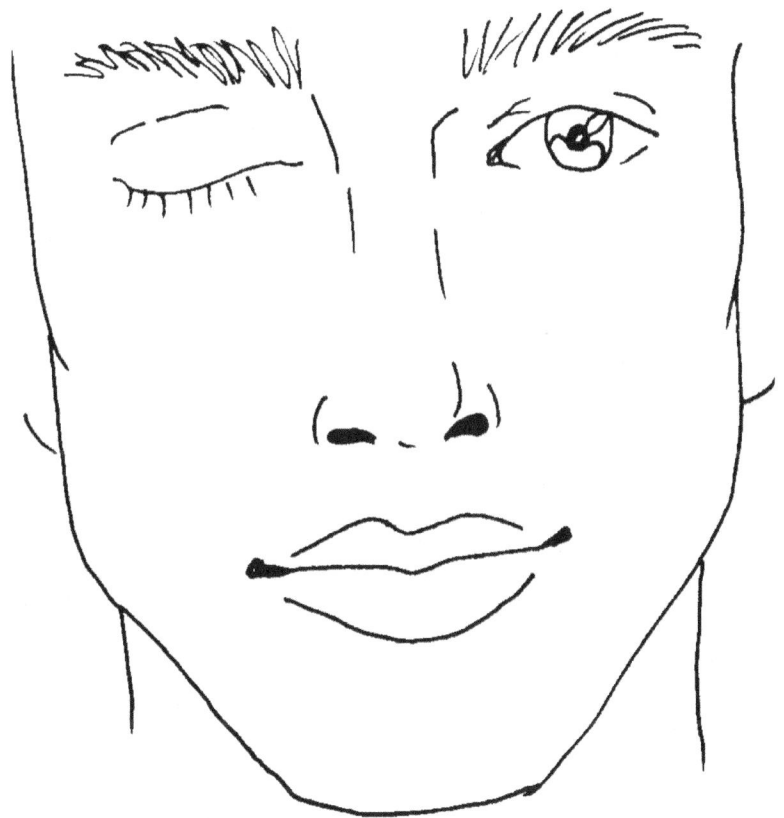

Face:

Primer:

Concealer:

Foundation:

Powder:

Blush:

Bronzer:

Contour:

Highlight:

Setting spray:

Facial Hair:

Inspiration:

Face/Body Paint:

Accessories:

Lips:

Liner:

Other:

Act Creation by Lara Johnson

If you want to get creative, you can even consider designing the hair of your character! This is not something I tend to draw out, but it is something I consider when putting my character together. It's also something that is affected by your props. If you have pigtails and do lots of spins, will they whack you in the face? Are you performing moves that will rely on your hair being out of your face? Is there a risk of your hair getting caught? Do you have amazing hair whips in your routine? Hair is sometimes a forgotten consideration. Whether you just think about it or sketch it to plan is up to you!

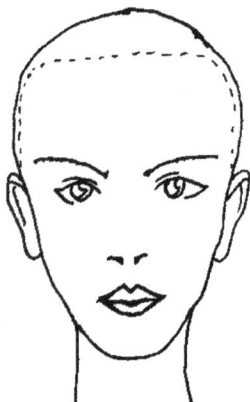

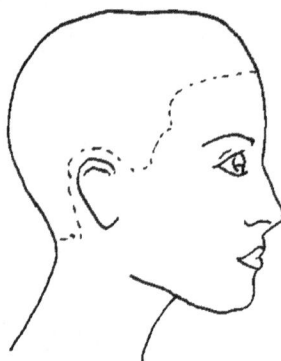

Option 1:

Notes:

_____
_____
_____
_____
_____

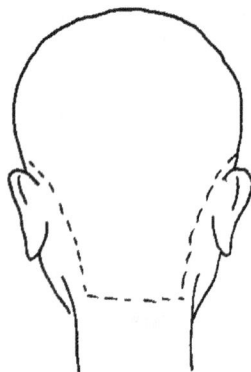

Option 2:

Notes:

_____
_____
_____
_____
_____

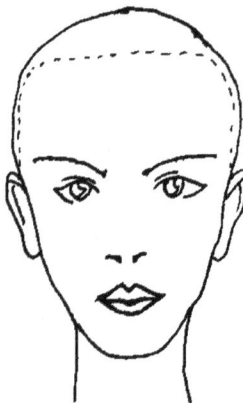

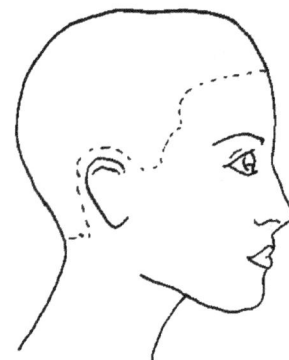

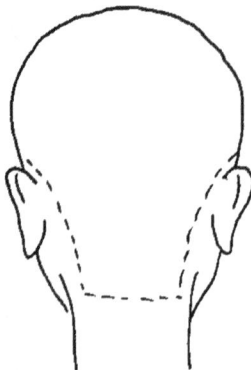

Hair Requirements:

_____
_____

Headdress/Hat requirements:

_____
_____

Notes about the image that I am wanting to create:

_____

_____

_____

_____

_____

_____

_____

_____

_____

_____

Feel free to add any images of inspiration here:

Tell Me About Yourself

Just like in school, when you filled out an "All about me" worksheet, here we will provide a brief snapshot of your character to refer back to.

Stage Name:

Character's Backstory:

Characters Personal Quirks:

Culture and Era, include any specific notes or requirements (if applicable):

Age and Gender Orientation notes (if applicable):

Relations and Reactions with Cast and Audience:

Costume Style:

Comfort/Movement Requirements:

Colours:

Other:

Hair and Makeup Notes:

Props and Accessories:

The next step is to work on visualising your look. This may change depending on your routine and move requirements. However, it is something that needs to be considered during the creation stage, as there may be certain props or items you need to add or remove throughout your journey. Visualisation is such a big thing. When you can see your character, it helps you see how they will act, walk, and move. This helps you feel the character and become the character onstage. Your look can change as your routine comes together, but it's great to have a rough idea to work towards.

Design and Visualise Your Costume

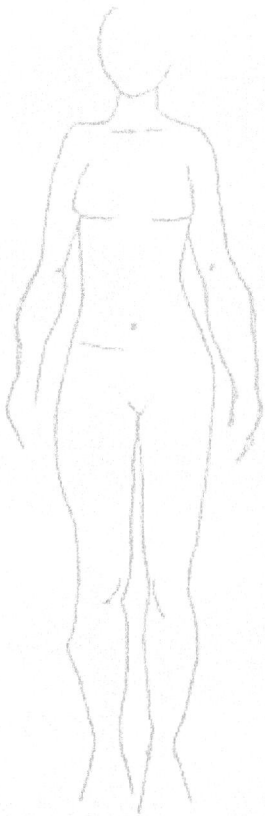

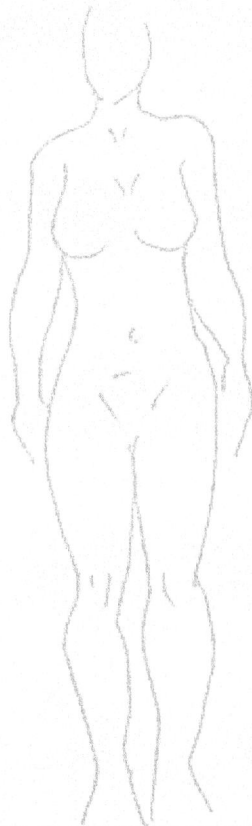

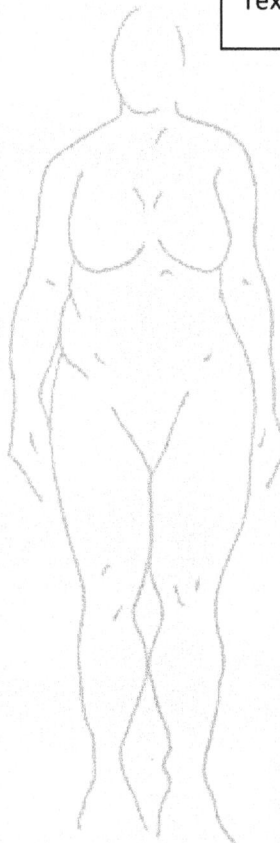

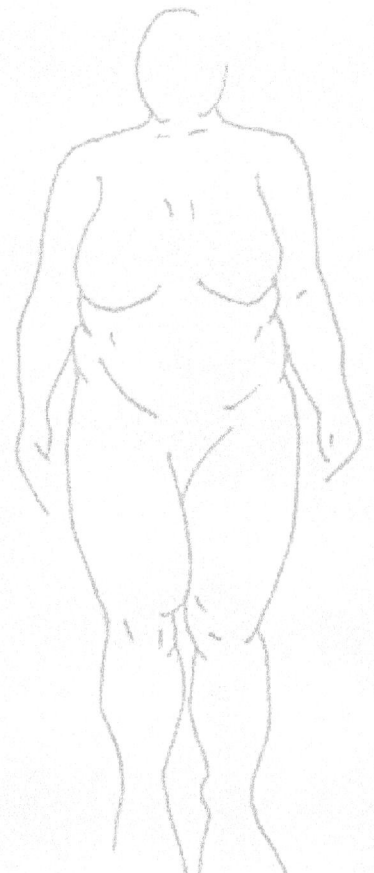

Costume Colour:

Top:

Bottom:

Highlight:

Costume Requirements:

Costume Fabric:

Type:

Texture:

Costume Accessories:

Footwear:

Jewellery:

Headwear:

Props or bags:

Shoes:

Other:

Design and Visualise Your Costume

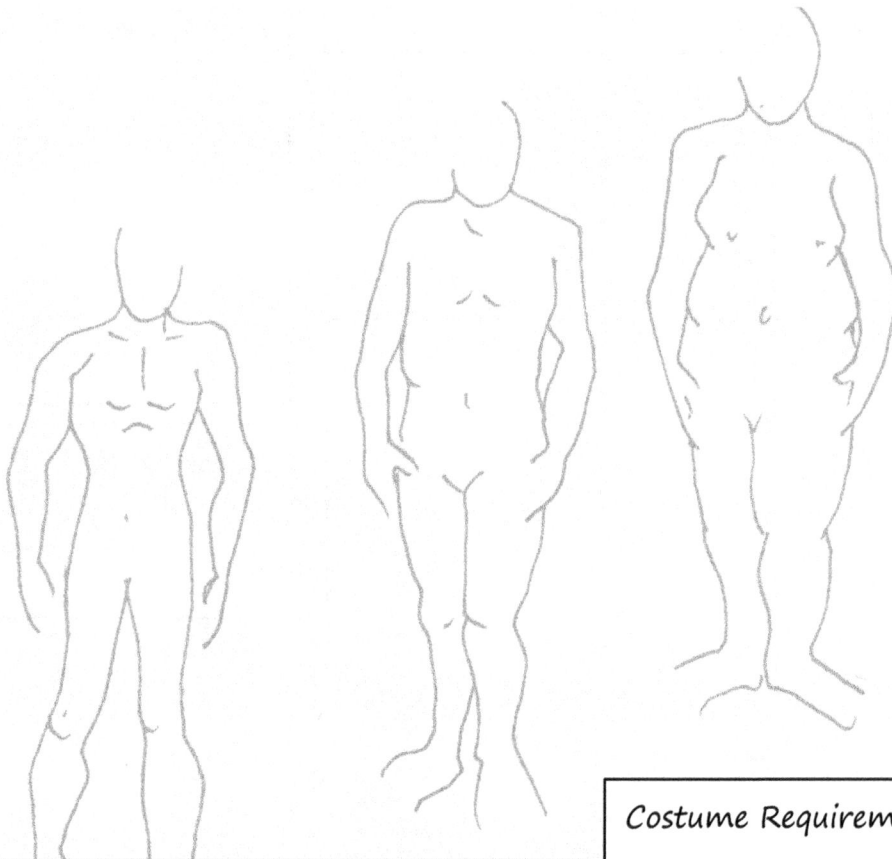

Costume Requirements:

Costume Colour:

Top:

Bottom:

Highlight:

Costume Accessories:

Footwear:

Jewellery:

Headwear:

Props or bags:

Shoes:

Other:

Costume Fabric:

Type:

Texture:

Draw or Collage

Use this space to draw or cut and paste pictures that inspire you. Choose images of costumes you like or words to consider with regard to your costume, including hair and makeup. Think about the look you want to create.

_____

_____

_____

_____

_____

_____

_____

_____

_____

_____

_____

_____

_____

_____

_____

_____

_____

_____

Do you have a costume designer? Make sure you note their contact details and deadline for completion. Have a little diary with notes, and fitting dates etc.

Prop Notes

Sometimes, when you think of a prop, you think of a whole range of things. You'll think about moves, risks, challenges, and more. This may be things you want to do, or things you shouldn't do. These elements sometimes get forgotten as you go through the routine. If you have a specific prop, sketch or list your ideas to get them out of your head and on paper before you forget about them.

_____

_____

_____

_____

_____

_____

_____

_____

_____

_____

Use this space to add pictures of any props you're considering or like the look and feel of.

Remember, your props must have a purpose. Every prop needs reason to be in your space and your act. How does it relate to your routine?

Act Creation by Lara Johnson

Performing

One thing you need to work out is if you are the act or if you are telling a story. You do not need to tell a story to perform a dance. It is an option, a focal point, but don't feel that it is necessary. People are coming to see you. You are the act, not the story, so you can flow and play to the music as you please.

This will vary depending on the theme and style of your act. For example, burlesque is about the build-up of tension, but it is also very much about telling a story. The narrative is important. The finale finishes off the routine, whether it is an amazing acro-balance or a particular trick. Your finale might be hula hoops swinging around your body or even a big reveal as you remove garments. It is light-hearted with larger-than-life expressions. Glamour, fantasy, and characterisation bring the audience in, and mystery captivates them. They may have both their hands showing, but they cannot wait for you to show yours, hiding beneath silky gloves.

With a story, you need to have an introduction, a climax, and a conclusion. In many dances, especially tease performances, the climax is the conclusion. However, don't forget the exit. The audience watches you walk onto the stage and leave it. You need to be confident in this too!

Use your space. I generally start a routine by introducing myself physically to the audience. I walk onstage in character and in routine. I use the space so that the audience feels involved and can see me. I then plan areas for certain moves. You don't want to be a dot at one spot on the stage. You want to make the most of the whole space. It is all there just for you to use... so use it! Be aware of any lights or other things that might restrict certain moves in certain areas. Whether it is in your way, or the stage item will restrict the audience's view of your performance. This is what your tech run is for!

Things to be aware of

If styling to align with a certain era, look at fashions, including clothes, hair, and makeup. Practise in your costume, and know how it influences the way you move.

Practising in costume is especially important if your performance involves the **removal of clothing**. Things like corsets can be awkward. Don't be afraid to ask the audience to get up and help if it's that type of environment. However, be aware that other people are not always reliable when it comes to looking after your costumes. Audience helpers might be nervous or try to show off in an unfamiliar environment. Be prepared. If it's not that type of environment, have a stagehand or a second person to assist you, and choreograph this process as part of your act so that it doesn't look like a mistake.

It can be valuable to know what type of flooring you're performing on ahead of time. If possible, ask the event organisers. Some floors are better for certain shoes, props, or fabrics. Some types might mean that you need to wear knee pads. Floor type has affected my choreography choices several times. You will also find that the type of footwear affects your choreography, again certain floor types may or may not allow for all types of footwear.

If you are doing an **aerial or pole performance**, it is also important to ensure that the height and space is appropriate and that you have a rigger sign off on the safety of the anchor points and the rigging itself. For **fire performers**, you need to consider not only liability and insurance requirements but also the size of the space. Can you create a safe barrier between you and the audience? How ventilated is the space, and are there any flammable risks around? You also need to know where the best and most secure fuel storage area is, as well as considering the location of your guarded fuelling bay. Don't forget about taps, fire extinguishers, and the location of your safety officer.

My notes:

_____

_____

_____

_____

_____

Removing Costuming

- **Zips** can get caught, so make sure that your costume is suitable and that nothing can get stuck in the zip. If using zips, it's best to make sure that there is not too much bulk. You also need to ensure that you're not going to awkwardly rest on your zip. Having all that pressure go through your pubic bone can be very uncomfortable!

- Feather **boas** leave a mess behind. Be wary if they are under costumes or tucked into pants, as you might look like you have hair where it doesn't belong. There are alternatives that look very effective and create less mess than feather boas. This will also help to look after animals a bit more than purchasing feathers! Have a look around, and see what options suit your act.

- If using **pop studs**, wear metal ones, and practise so that you know how they move and that they won't pop while you're performing.

- If taking off **garter belts**, a layer of undies, or anything similar, remember you will need to slide them off the heel, then over the toe of your shoes.

- **Velcro** only works for large-scale shows. In smaller environments, audiences can hear it rip and sometimes see it, which ruins the effect.

- Don't forget that if **stockings** are being rolled down, you'll need to take your shoes off first. Also consider the gusset of the stocking. Sometimes, this can look pretty shocking, so look around for slimline gussets that don't stand out at all. I generally wear these under everything to make my legs look seamless, even under fishnets or other stockings. If you're having problems with your stockings getting static or sticking to your legs, try to moisturise and shave prior to putting them on. This helps them glide. Ensure that your nails are freshly filed so that you don't nick them on your stockings and cause rips or tears. Any ladders can be emergency halted with clear nail polish. If you have dry skin, you can also moisturise your hands before performing to prevent skin from getting caught on stockings. Make sure you have rehearsed in your stockings with high heels, as they feel quite different to walk in. If your stockings start sliding down too soon, use two flat palms to guide them up again.

- **Buttons** are awkward! If you're wearing gloves, you will learn that nothing is easy, and everything is seemingly impossible. Practise, practise, practise. Differently sized and shaped buttons all have their pros and cons. Get used to how your buttons work.

- **Bows** are fabulous, but they do carry a risk of getting caught or slipping undone. Satin is renowned for this. If you want to tie your costume up in a bow, make sure that you aren't going to get stuck and accidentally undo it too early.
- Be aware of how you're taking things off. Make it look pretty, and drag it out. There's no need to rush. Keep it classy and elegant by not pulling things inside out, especially if they have tags. Tags and seams really detract from what you're doing, and it looks much less sophisticated to have everything inside out onstage!
- Remove tags! The worst look is to have a big tag showing in your costume, either sticking out the back or visible when you take it off. Make life easier for yourself, and remove the tag before you perform.

Practice makes everything a lot easier, which means that almost nothing is impossible.

My notes:

_____

_____

_____

_____

_____

_____

_____

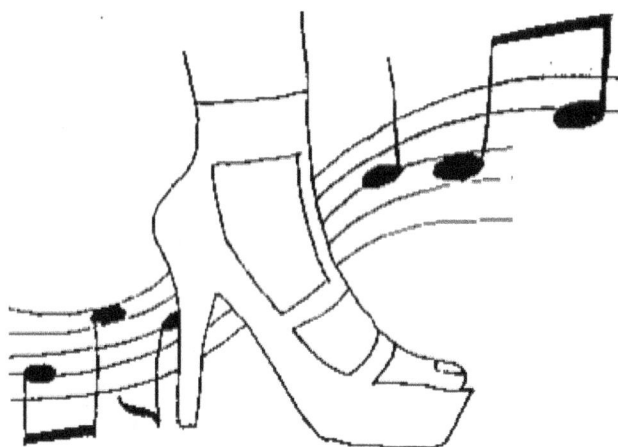

Creating Choreography

When it comes to creating choreography, it really does depend on how your head works. Are you a storyteller? Is it all about the visual elements? What about the feeling, the moves, the flow, or the music? Everyone is different. But here are a few tips that may help you on your way.

If you think about steps for creating choreography, it looks a little like the list below, except the first two steps are slightly interchangeable. Some people start with the music, which inspires them to create an act, a character, or a theme. Others start with an idea, and they create an act based on that idea, character, theme, or story. Neither method is wrong. It is your journey of creation. But these elements are usually among the first in the journey to create an act.

1. Choose a theme and character.

2. Choose a song. Part of choosing your song is getting to know the song. Understand how it works by breaking down all the little parts and components of it. Identifying these helps you to work out where movements should go. Is your music flowy, or are there dramatic moments?

3. Personally, I theme my routines around the song and then build the character based on this. I know many other performers who do this too. Every now and then, you have an idea that you want to build from scratch, which is when you break down your theme and character first. Many people new to performing find that knowing their character helps them choose music that suits. This is just a guide. Use the order that works best for you.

4. It's time to play! See what feels good. Record it, and consider what looks good. Play with the sections that feel right for you, in no particular order. This way you can chunk out your song so that you can join it all together later on! Take lots of notes and videos, and practise on repeat. You will notice that some sections of the song feel right or like they need a certain style of movement. Block them out, and make a note of this.

5. Next, look at linking these sections and sequences together. Start to fill in the gaps with your transitions and other moves. You can find a natural flow, or you can find something completely different. Practise until it feels natural. Or you can find a natural flow, and as you get used to it, you can elaborate and build on it to give it more depth.

6. After this, it's all about practice, just like on show night, in character! This way, you'll know your routine inside out, which will help you deal with any unexpected events on show night with ease.

Now that you know your structure, there are some things you can do to improve further.

1. Don't feel like you need to start at the start. Allow your routine to flow by starting wherever you're inspired. This will feel like you're choreographing the easiest part first. It allows you to feel the flow of how the song works for you. If you have a combination you want to use, start with that and work around it. Things don't need to be chronological. They just have to get there in the end!

    I personally print my song's lyrics, and I time-map them. I colour-code them to show where the beat changes or where there is a difference in music or style. If this is repeated, like a chorus, then all of these elements are the same colour. This helps me see how the music flows without constantly pressing stop and start. I then build on it, block by block.

    If you are a storyteller, you can draw a story board. Find a way to put your ideas on paper or in your body. Make sure you record what you have done so that you don't forget it! It is the worst feeling to find the perfect flow and forget what it was. This is why I divide the routine into blocks. Otherwise, I come back after a run-through and find that don't remember what the first few transitions were.

2. You don't have to do it all at once! Hack away at your routine a little bit at a time. Give yourself a deadline, and work on it slowly. As long as you're making progress, you're on the right track. Ensure that you stick to your deadline, and balance your training so that you don't fatigue. Some sessions might just involve stepping your routine through or working on transitions. Others can focus on the big combinations. If you have a prop, train with it, and get used to how it moves. This is all about understanding how you choreograph, so get comfortable with your own style, and be aware of what you may need to adjust to make it work. Creating balance in your schedule helps big time. Don't force someone else's method of choreography. That will block your creativity, as you will feel restricted. Do what works for you!

3. Flow with your inspiration. Once you get inspired, move with it, and go as far as you feel comfortable without adding extra restrictions on time or transitions. It isn't easy to achieve a state of flow, so use it when you have it!

4. You can also think of your routine as a pizza or a lasagne. Either way, it has layers. Each section has layers. You can train a section of your routine until it is so natural to you that the moves no longer feel tricky or intense. From here, you can add character to them or increase the depth of your movement. You can add other flourishes or make them trickier. Your routine grows with you, and as you begin to find it easier, you can add complexities. If you want a multi-layered and complex show, you don't have to start with that. You can layer it on.

5. People talk about writer's block, and you can also get dancer's block. Don't get too stuck on ideas. Let go of them if you're feeling restricted, and see where things can flow to. Maybe your mindset will be different. A routine is a living thing, so give it life, and let it breathe, live, and evolve. It is a changeable process, not limited by restrictions (unless they are there for safety reasons).

6. Videos are awesome! You can record your session and go back later to review it. How does it flow? How do the lines work? What about the transitions? Pull your routine apart, and piece your next training session together using the notes you have taken away from your last one.

7. Remember to analyse your music. Find out what story it is telling, considering the emotion and feeling that it evokes. Music isn't just about beat and rhythm. You want to tell a story through your movements. At the same time, you want to make your routine imaginative and unique. Whether you use technique, rhythm, or style, make it you. Remember that when you tell a story, there should be an introduction, a climax, and a conclusion. This is also the case in dance. Build up to the wow moments, and don't just taper the dance off. Finish it with a bang!

8. If music isn't your thing and listening to lyrics doesn't work, many routines are choreographed with movements to a count of 8. Feel free to break your routine down into counts if this is helpful for you.

9. Stuck with a few chunks and not sure how to piece them together? Get out of your head, and put the music on. Freestyle the movement. See what your body is inspired to do.

10. Be aware of your space. How much room do you have to perform? What is the area like? Where is your audience? Ensure that your moves end facing the direction that you want them to. Use all of your space! Your stage isn't just the dot where you stand, so play, interact, or at least acknowledge the audience, and use your space. Don't forget to consider what else you can bring to your space, including lighting, sound effects, and visual effects. How can you take the extra step with what is available to you? If you are using these things, they must have a purpose, and they must fit with the story you're telling, helping to create a fuller picture for the audience. These elements should draw on emotion and be involved in your story.

11. Feel free to watch other performers, and see what inspires you. This is part of fuelling your inspiration. I find it so motivating to see what can be done. Look at different styles of movement or dance, and see if you can incorporate some of these elements in your routine. Do some research, and see what comes from it. Remember, not everything has to have the extreme wow factor. When put together seamlessly, basics are beautiful and amazing.

12. Many people are offended by frontal thrusts and spreads. These can be seen to be too crude for some environments and dance styles. You can do similar movements to other angles to create tension with concealment. Work out what your audience demographic is before looking at these moves. Will there be families? Is your routine appropriate if there are children in the audience, or will you perform at an adult-only event? Even traditional burlesque was about the tease, not full-frontal motions. Much of burlesque is about curves, making them big in one area and small in another.

My notes:

_____

_____

_____

_____

_____

_____

_____

_____

_____

_____

_____

Do your moves make sense to the story and music that you are telling? Or are they contradictory? Once you have started to piece things together go over it and make sure your moves, concept and music all align. Remember stories follow a format, they have their introduction, then they build to have their climax, sometimes the climax is the end, other times it comes back down to finish, but plan the three parts, introduction, body and conclusion so that it doesn't feel odd to the audience to suddenly be finishes.

Elements of Dance

Keep the basic elements of dance in mind when choreographing, even breaking moves down into patterns, styles, and footwork. You can use one of these elements as part of your focus.

Work out what your strengths are and what comes easily to you. This should be your initial focus. Otherwise, you're just making things harder for yourself. You want to balance your strengths with your weaknesses to get a sense of adjustments you may need to make. For example, you may be flexible but bad at timing, or you might use space fantastically but be one-sided in your movements. You may be able to create amazing shapes but not know how to use them. Being aware of your strengths and weaknesses will help you piece together a routine and give you awareness of what you need to adjust.

Space:

Think about the way you move through and interact with your space. This is the way you occupy your little world onstage. You can look at actual movement or direction of movement and implied movement in the form of placements and gestures. Consider dynamic levels and your relationship not only to the floor and the pole but also to the sky. The space isn't just the place where you stand; it's the air above you too. You need to look at the size of your moves. Are they big or small? What is your orientation? Where do you need to face? Where is the pole, and where are any props, other performers, and even the audience? What is your relationship to these elements or people?

Time:

Time is generally set by the music's rhythm and tempo. Your movements can make some of these musical rhythms seem bigger or almost obsolete. You can do everything to the beat or completely against it. Find your sense of rhythm, and develop it. Once you have found it, maintain it throughout the whole dance, or have obvious points in your routine where this changes. How else can you look at time? Quite literally, by the clock! How do your movements align with those of other performers? Have bit of fun, and be unpredictable. Play with a completely free rhythm, relying on cues from other performers instead of the music.

Form or Shape:

Form and shape can take a number of paths and can really be two different categories. Focus on perfection of form and lines, from your fingertips down to your toes. Alternatively, you could embody the shape of an animal. Think of the body as a mobile figure. You create shapes that evoke a feeling in you, and this is what the audience sees. You can have different shapes that you create. They can be twisted or symmetrical, but the important part is what your body does to lead into this movement and out of it. Dance is not just the position itself but the road that gets you there! The shapes you create onstage will differ depending on the style of your routine or the props you use. Even a breath can be an important moment in a routine. Internally, you have ideas, identity, intention, and emotion. This comes out in the form of expression and communication. You want to find the balance of moving through these, inviting the audience into your story.

Force and Energy:

Even if you have two people onstage and they use their timing and space in the same way, they can look completely different in terms of the energy, force, and emotion they put into their performance. You can do the same thing but in a slack, depressed persona, and it would look very different to the performance of someone having the time of their life. What energy or feelings do you want to evoke through your movements? You can also look at energy by considering things with weight. Are you performing a heavy motion, or are your movements light and flowy? Is it a sharp, sudden movement or a more sustained and smoother motion? What is the flow and quality of your movement?

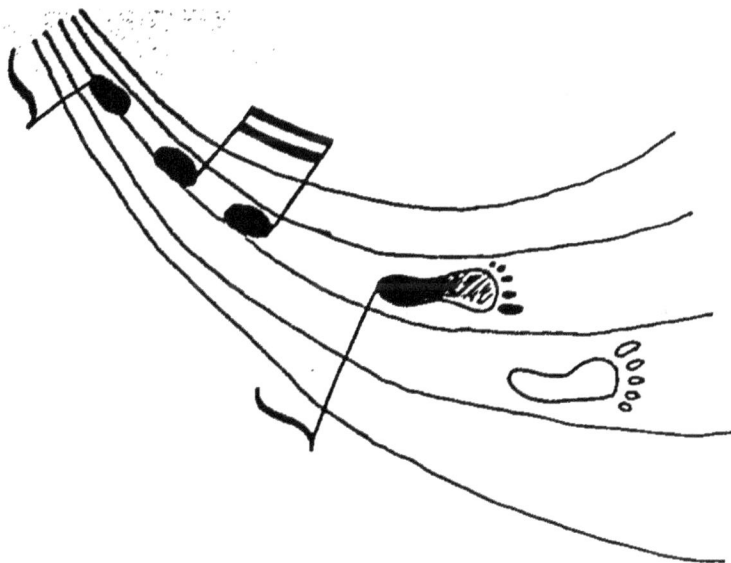

Make training fun, and enjoy the process. If you enjoy it, others are bound to as well. So often, things are overthought. It's important get out of your head and into your body. Once you have the general structure, you can get back into your head to analyse movements and perfect your form, lines, flow, and transitions. This is when you can improve whatever you need to work on. The heart and body come first, the head second!

Write down what struck you about creating choreography so that you can remember it in the future.

_____

_____

_____

_____

_____

_____

_____

_____

_____

_____

_____

_____

Sketch any ideas that this section inspired.

When learning choreography, having a note pad to write down little cues, transitions, or even intentions of movement can help to organise your thoughts and feel confident about what you are doing. It can feel very overwhelming putting together a performance, but having little notes can help slowly make it feel more manageable.

Inspiration Notes

(The pole aspects are purely to look at stylistic differences, and differences in levels/height. If you are doing another artform, you can still use these elements, just re-word them)

Characterisation quirks:

Floor-to-pole moves:

Floor moves:

Up-the-pole moves:

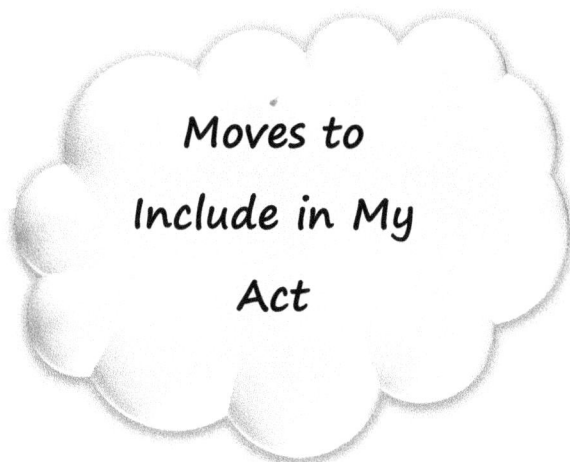

Moves to Include in My Act

Inversions:

Pole spins:

Dismounts:

Cool transitions:

Signature poses:

Act Creation by Lara Johnson

Music Choice

Music Style:

Meaning behind the music:

_____

_____

What the music means to me:

_____

_____

_____

_____

Feeling the music evokes:

_____

_____

Why I chose it:

_____

_____

_____

Favourite lyrics:

_____

_____

Words or lyrics that match certain movements:

_____

_____

Tone and pace of the song:

_____

_____

Map Your Song

I map out my music with timestamps and lyrics, then list the moves I want to use. This way, I can choreograph the parts of the song that inspire me most. If you are musical, you can do this with sheet music, choreographing to specific musical notes. I outline the things I think should go in certain spots, then fill in the gaps. I also colour code or mark out the different tones, sounds, changes in beat or chorus so that I can map my moves to match the musicality of my song.

Dance Genre:
Date:
Song Name:
Artist:

Timestamp	Lyrics	Moves I Want Here

I then colour-code parts of the song where the music repeats or changes, and I identify the chorus. This means that I can map out which moves need to be repeated. I can also see at a glance where I am up to in my routine.

Please be cautious of cultural song choices. Ensure that you look into any tradition or meaning behind a cultural or traditional piece of music before putting together your act. The last thing you want is to be disrespectful or offend anyone by putting the wrong style show to a particular piece of music.

Song Related Notes:

_____

_____

_____

_____

_____

_____

_____

_____

_____

_____

_____

_____

_____

_____

What is the general feel of the song, and how does this relate to your movements? Do you have any personal experienced which this song reminds you of, that gives you a personal link to the music? It isn't necessary, but if you do, you can use that to your advantage!

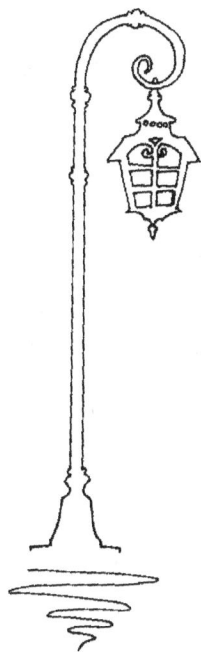

As the audience sits in silent anticipation, the curtains draw back to reveal a lone streetlamp in the middle of the otherwise empty stage. It flickers with a gentle orange glow. Suddenly, out of nowhere, the lights flash like lightning as you enter, holding an umbrella. There is a moment of confusion, as you are not on the stage. You are noticed by some, and a nudge of acknowledgement goes through the audience as each person lets the next know where you are. You appear through the back of the audience, dodging the storm as you traipse down the aisles and towards the stage. The audience turns and looks around to see what is happening, their eyes following you as you climb the stairs to the stage. A warm glow of light fills the room like the sun has returned. And the act has begun.

Setting the Stage

Setting the stage is all about the effective use of space. The aim is **for your space to enhance the performance**, to create a focal point. You can even add in some of your branding! How you set the stage will depend on your budget and any technology requirements, as well as any customisation or branding inclusions. If you are performing for someone else, you need to consider the time it takes to set up and pack down the stage. If you are setting up a big show for others to perform, this needs to be taken into account for every act.

You want to consider safety and access, as well as the time required to set up, pack down, and perform. If you have props, you want them to be lightweight and versatile so that they are easy to move. You want to be able to use the entire stage, blocking out where specific actions are going to go. As you do so, you need to ensure that you are in a good line of sight and aren't blocking the audience's view with props and lighting. You also want to ensure that you aren't doing floorwork next to the stage lighting. This ensure that you won't be blocked or blinded by the light! Consider your act from the audience's point of view. Remember that the stage height may also come into play with some moves and detract from the view of the audience.

When you start out as a performer, you may not be in charge of the visual setup of the stage. You may be provided with a stage space to perform on, and you will need to bring any props with you when you are ready to perform. If you need someone to do this for you, make sure you communicate that you would like your prop to be centre stage before you come on.

If you have **electrical items** in your act, you also need to consider where the nearest power outlet will be, and you'll need to tape down any electrical cords to avoid tripping hazards. Ensure that the venue is okay with you using tape, as some places, such as heritage buildings, may have restrictions on certain things. Ask what's available for you to use. Some venues even have carpet designed to cover cords!

Remember that around a stage, there is **always movement** of MCs, stagehands, and other performers. Keep this in mind when putting together your stage design so that you don't block pathways. This is especially important if there is rigging or something else that requires access during the show. The good news is that decluttering also helps to maintain focus, immersing your audience in the experience.

You want to look at the **visual composition** of the stage. Consider the lines you create with your props, and avoid blocking the view of the audience. Consider how large and small items are arranged onstage to create balance. You want cohesion. Things need to go together so that they are not a mismatched mess. Choose elements that align with your act's theme and the event's goals so that these things do not conflict. Colour, shape, style, and texture are all things to consider if setting an elaborate stage. Texture can feel like an odd addition, but it can provide depth and visual interest.

Fortunately, dancers usually have minimal props to consider. Instead, focus on how you space and balance items on the stage. You need to consider other **outside elements**, like microphones. Are you using a microphone? Is it on a cord or a stand? Where is it placed? You also need to consider any white space, ensuring that you balance the space you have and don't leave one section empty. Look at where you will move. Can you create repetition in your staging? Allow for movement, and ensure the environment is balanced and in proportion.

Another thing you need to consider is **lighting**. Lighting sets mood, which you can add to with your energy and movements. So much of a good performance begins with lighting elements. Be aware of people who may be triggered by flashing lights, as this can detract from your performance. In some instances, flashing may create a great panic effect on the stage, but it can cause issues in the audience. Don't just think outside the box; think outside the stage! It isn't your only space. Depending on the setup of the event, you may be able to do something different.

Let's simplify all of this information.

You want things simple and balanced. If you dress the side of the stage with props, this will make your space appear larger and may help to draw the audience's attention to the centre. Check every technical detail, and ensure you're not creating trip hazards in your show. Allow time to set up and pack down, and consider this when choosing props. If you have aerial props, check for vertical shapes or hanging lights, as well as your ceiling height.

If you are on a small stage, you can use large props or elements to deliver an impact. Just make sure that your props don't block or detract from your performance. If a prop doesn't enhance your performance, don't use it. Use the space, and consider the audience's point of view.

Elements to Consider in Your Space:

- audio/visual equipment
- furniture
- lighting
- set décor and props
- stage height

- audience blind spots

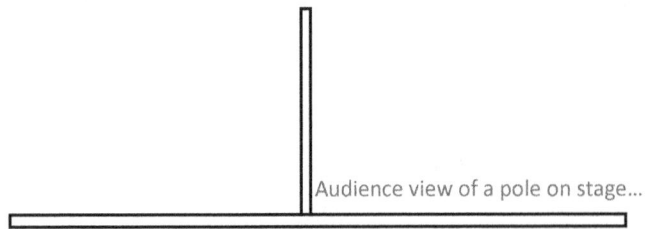

- access.

Your Stage Should:

- be simple and uncluttered

- have clear lines of sight

- be safe and accessible

- draw focus to your act.

Audience view of a pole on stage…

Aerial view of a pole on stage…

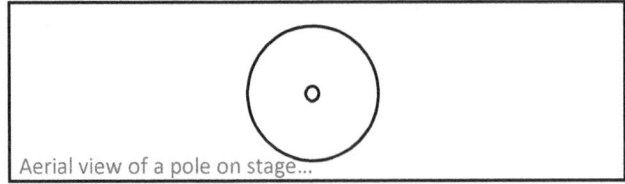

This allows you to map where your moves can be on stage, to make sure the space is used evenly and efficiently.

I recommend "stage mapping" draw out your stage, and mark on there where your props will be in the space to make sure you are using your space evenly. This can be done from a birds eye view, like you are looking down from on the stage from the air. I would then "block" out your movements on the stage. This will allow you to ensure that you are using the whole stage in your performance. Even if it is just "I am using this general area when on the floor" and another general area for a particular prop. This helps you see where all your movements are going to be, not only so that you personally can visualise and feel confident with where you are going in space. But also, so that you can ensure that you are utilising your entire stage effectively.

My notes:

_____

_____

_____

_____

_____

_____

_____

Stage Directions

When you're setting up a stage or asking people to put things on the stage, there are a few things that are helpful to know. Directions of right and left are communicated from the performer's point of view, not the audience's perspective. Upstage is the back of the stage. Downstage is the front or audience-side of the stage. Centre stage is in the middle. I tend to think of how many stages are raised from the audience, so where the audience sits, is known as downstage.

Upstage right	Upstage centre	Upstage left
Centre stage right	Centre stage	Centre stage left
Downstage right	Downstage centre	Downstage left
Audience		

Types of Stages

There are a few main types of stage. There are more, but this covers the majority of stage types you will get to know throughout your performing journey. Each stage type offers a different sightline, as well as prop and backdrop considerations. Think of the audience. They could be on one, two, three, or four side of the stage. Here are the main stage types you should know.

- Thrust: I think of this one as a poky stage. Generally, there is a rectangular stage and audiences on three of the sides of the stage. You can still have a backdrop, but this stage type makes you feel like you can go out into the audience while remaining on the stage.

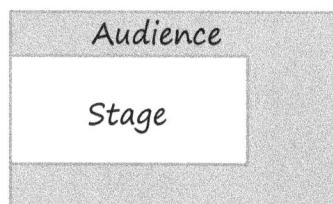

- Arena: In an arena, you are on a stage in the middle of the crowd. Here, you have no background, and you need to interact and perform on all sides of the stage. An arena stage may be circular or squared.

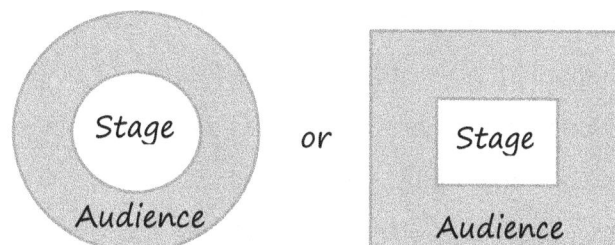

- Found: This stage type is just what it sounds like. It is a place that is found and turned into a stage. Generally, audiences are seated in front of the stage, but this is not always the case. The use of props, lighting, and other technical elements will be more minimalistic with this stage type.

- Traverse: This is a stage setup that we don't often see in our art form, but it is an option nonetheless. A traverse stage seats audiences on two sides, so you need to be careful not to face your back to either side for too long. You need to design the routine so that audiences are facing each side of you or so that the back-facing elements are included in your artistic design and choreography. Set design for traverse staging is much more limited, as props can easily block view.

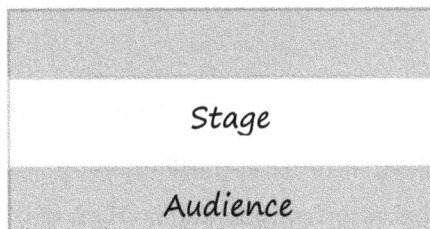

- Proscenium: If you go to the theatre and see a big stage with curtains or an old-school arch, this is a proscenium stage. Generally, these stages have the front of the stage, visible to the audience, and side stages in the wings to help get items on and off. Often, there is also a deep stage to play with. There is not necessarily an orchestral pit, but you may be lucky enough to have one!

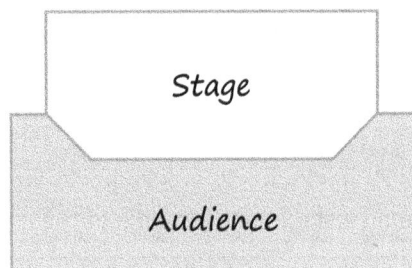

Finally, there are mobile or outdoor stages. Here, you need to consider wind, sun, and weather. Does sunscreen make you slippery, or do some moves suffer in the wind? The direction the stage is facing becomes important, as you need to ensure that no one on or off the stage is squinting into the sun. Surrounding distractions will also need to be taken into account. You need to consider acoustics and how sound works and travels. The size of the stage may also limit the number of performers. Outdoors, you can use natural focal points around you to create a backdrop for your performance.

A Personal Anecdote

I once performed a show where we only had a few minutes to confirm the tech and everything else before going onstage. I had sent in my music and had everything organised, so I was quite confident. I went over to the tech person to confirm that they were happy with my song and the point where I wanted it to stop. They said yes but put the song on at the point where it should have ended. It was the wrong part of the music! I told the tech the music cue, and we adjusted it on the system. I thought it was strange, but I walked away feeling grateful that I'd checked. Otherwise, I would have been stuck halfway through my routine. What I didn't know was that the tech people had put another version of the song on the list instead of the version I'd sent through. They thought it was the same, only louder, allowing it to work better with their setup.

I got onstage as the first act, and within seconds, I knew my song was a different version. It had talking. It had instrumentals. It had singing. Even the order in which the song told its story was different. There I was, having just started my routine, which at that point included standing choreography. But the part of the music the show had started with was supposed to be for floorwork. Everything was reversed. Suddenly, I had no idea how long the track was going to last, what would come next, or how I was going to progress.

My natural reaction was to try to adjust my movements and keep up with the music, but the music was more different than I had feared. I shut the music out of my mind and continued. I knew the story my movements were going to tell. I decided to tell that story and feel the music as I went to see if I needed any more climactic or dramatic moves to make it appear more seamless. I performed my routine and no one knew what a challenge it had been. I had a tight feeling in my chest, and my head felt like it was floating. I did it. I made it! It was fun and a little stressful, but I did it! Learning to adapt was the key.

Things to Consider When Performing

Much of this list is related to burlesque, but these considerations can be applied across many styles of dance.

- Look at the audience, and if it suits your character, give cheeky or emotive looks back constantly. Audience interaction isn't always overt. This will depend on your act and character. If you look slightly above the audience, over their heads, you will give the illusion that you are looking at more people.

- Don't be afraid. Many performers wouldn't dare do what their character does. They are not that person, but their character is. Remember that your character is not a reflection of you.

- Don't be afraid to touch. Whether it's your prop or yourself, use your senses. Use your hands to trace your side or play with your hair. Make each movement count. You can emphasise your senses and create situations that your audience can relate to.

- Facial expressions are essential. They really finish off your routine. This is important, so practise until you know your routine well, then play when performing it. This helps to relax your concentration face.

- Ruffle your hair if it suits your character. It's a part of you too, and many people would love to run their fingers through it. Make them envious.

- Remember that emotion influences your movement. Whatever emotion you are trying to portray should also be in your posture, your steps, and the way you flow. Bring emotion into your performance.

- If you mess up, play on it. Make someone fix it, or use it as a prop or an opportunity for audience participation. No one else knows you made a mistake if you don't try to cover it up! As long as a movement is purposeful, it is seen as correct!

- Lip glosses can run, so be careful with your makeup choices.

- Do a lap of the stage within the first 45 seconds of your choreography before commencing the routine. This is your introduction and can be choreographed. Stay in character, and use eye contact. Don't be afraid to interact, and thank your audience at the end of your performance.

- If you're in a bad mood, do the routine as if you are. Harshly rip off your gloves or whatever you're removing, and include this tone in your movements. Don't try and fake a mood. Using your current mood can help to ensure you don't get typecast as a certain character. It doesn't have to be all about glitz and glam. You can create your character and world onstage.

- Risqué arts, like burlesque and pole dancing, don't have to be all about the removal of clothing. If you want to do it, you can try making the removal look like an accident. Make your audience invest in your choreography so that they don't notice clothing being removed until it is gone. Alternatively, removal can be a dragged-out feature. Burlesque can include all levels of satire and unusual arts, from hooping to fire and go-go dancing. You can tell different stories using different styles of technical dance and different types of movements and flow. You don't have to do or be what many may expect.

- If you're dealing with troublesome hecklers in the audience, use your character to shoo them off, or bring one onstage to tame them. Being careful to not put yourself at risk or offend the audience member. This is a risky move, as you never know how they will react or what may trigger or offend. But it is an option nonetheless.

- Things are always different when you have a live audience. The feeling is different, the reaction is different, and the environment is different. Sometimes, it helps just to be aware of that!

I have a friend who performs regularly, and one thing that really threw her once was lighting. She walked onstage, and there was no difference between stage lighting and audience lighting. You could see everyone. It really hit her as she walked out, and it took her a few moments to recalibrate.

But you are onstage. You know your act, and the world you create becomes your focus. Mishaps and unexpected adventures may happen. If you know your act well enough, you can bring yourself back to the moment. Focus on your routine and the onstage world you are creating. You can mentally prepare by knowing your routine and being confident in your abilities. This saves some of your thinking space to deal with uh-oh moments before you bring yourself back to the task at hand. Sometimes, if you are mid-performance, you can react to a mishap and make it look like it was part of your routine. This gives you a few moments to bring yourself back in and continue.

I think one of the most important lessons of this section that applies to any performance style is that only you know your routine. **If you do something wrong, no one else knows!** Don't make a fuss of it. Pretend it was supposed to be there, and carry on.

Movement

- Each movement is tantalising. It has a purpose, so make the most of it!

- Moves are like a language. You want to use your moves and motions to communicate with those watching. The smoother your transitions are, the more your story will make sense and the more you'll retain the interest of your audience.

- There is always a new way of moving that you haven't done before. Something new you can do with your body in relation to movement. Exploring new and unusual pathways can unlock new flow and different unique transitions.

- Use a mix of levels. Stand, kneel, sit, lie, and make the most of the area. Do moves up the pole, then some low on the pole. Include some spins and some floorwork. Dynamic levels generate interest in your routine. The great thing about a pole is that it adds to the space you can use. You don't just have the stage; you have the sky too!

- Watch where your hands are going. This is where the audience will look, so hand placement is important.

- Play with the order of your tricks or moves. Mix and match the order of your steps and tricks to create an opportunity for amazing flow and transitions. This can provide different levels of anticipation for the audience. You don't always want to be predictable. A flow that feels exact can sometimes get lost. Moving it can create a whole new way of looking at moves. Consider different motions, and change the way the audience sees your routine.

- Plan for your style and the expected demographic of your show's audience.

- Listen to your song and its lyrics. Understand the song, and choreograph as if you are a part of the song. You could be the cheater, the cheated, the heartbreaker, the frustrated friend, and so on.

- On large stages, your character must fill the room. The bigger the space, the bigger the character must be. You don't want to just be a dot on the stage!

- Remember that you don't have to use every trick or even your favourite tricks or moves. Flow with what works for your character and the feel of the routine, but don't get typecast as always doing the same moves and combinations. If you always use the same tricks or the same ways in or out of a move, your performance can get boring. I like to pick a different focal move for a climax moment in the routine. I build up to the move and use the trick in different ways. This opens new doors for movement that I may not have previously considered. Making it more interesting not only for the audience, but for the performer too!

- I really enjoy linking heaven and Earth movements going up and down. This uses space and creates balance and interest in routines. It stops everything from being so upward and balances it with an opposite. This doesn't have to be completely literal. You can do a fingertip trail up, while down movements may come from the feet. Use your whole body, and play with the notion that what comes up must go down. Once you are at the bottom, the only way is up. This can be any element of the body or any type of feeling or movement. If you're getting stuck with flow of movement, it's a good thing to consider.

- If you're doing a group performance, it's a good idea to look at rotations of the front and back lines. Choreograph this into your movements. This ensures that no one feels like they are always stuck at the back or always front and centre. Choreograph to suit everyone's strengths, and create new positions for people to move to so that everyone gets a fair share of the limelight.

- Can you achieve all the moves you want to in your costume? Can you do the splits if needed? In burlesque, are there gems that could get caught? In pole, do you have all your grip points? In fire, are you wearing natural fibres and non-flammable thread? These are important safety considerations.

- Whenever you perform, remember to breathe through your moves!

- Moves can be changed just by adding your own flair, am arm movement, a leg angle, make them different, uniquely you!

- Use the music to highlight your tricks, you can look so much more dramatic, or enhanced if you use the music in such a way that it enhances your movement.

My notes:

_____

_____

_____

_____

_____

_____

_____

Planes of Movement

The body has three planes of movement. Creating and promoting movement in all of these planes or staying within specific planes for certain movements helps to add depth to your routine. The three planes are the frontal, sagittal, and transverse planes.

- Frontal: This one is pretty straightforward. Think of movements that can be seen fully and completely in front of you. Imagine the body being divided between front and back. If you spin or do other circus things, this is also sometimes referred to as the wall plane, as if you were facing a wall. I remember which one by thinking "F" for front, and thus frontal.

- Sagittal: This plane is more sideways focused. It is a movement that can be seen side-on. Remember being a kid and pretending to be on a bus or train with your hands at your side like wheels? This is the sagittal plane. Many performers, especially those who do object manipulation, refer to the sagittal plane as the wheel plane. I remember which one by thinking "S" for side, "S" for sagittal.

- Transverse: Picture a high-waisted tutu going around your body and dividing it in half. There is the top and the bottom. This is the transverse plane. Sometimes, this is referred to as the horizontal plane. From a performance point of view, it may help to think of this as a lasso action, a flat spin up or down. I remember which one by thinking "T" for top or tutu, "T" for Transverse.

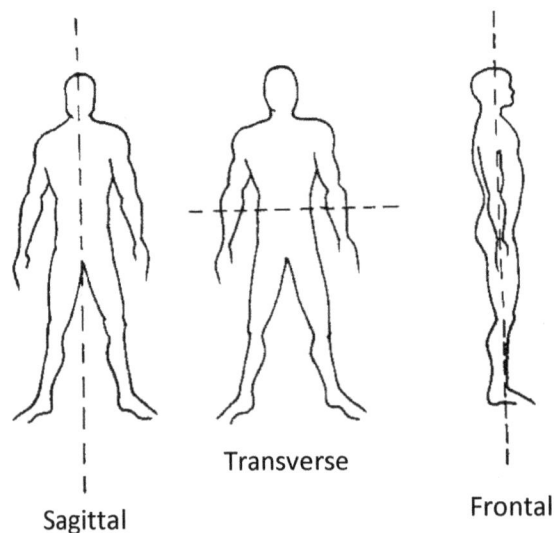

Sagittal   Transverse   Frontal

Hand Movements

Hand choreography is its own genre. Hand motions can vary from wave movements to hitting movements, flipping motions, and intricate finger movements. There is so much that a hand can say, which is one reason why many cultures communicate with hand gestures.

Holding something tight can represent tension. Suggestively running your hand over something tells its own story. They finish the line of our arm, so if you want a straight line, that line or energy also needs to flow all the way out through your fingertips. Regardless, hands need a purpose wherever they are, whether they're walking, resting on a prop, aiding in interaction, or presenting to the audience. Be aware of what your hands are saying and where they are. Hands are important, and they can also be distracting. They need to be used to draw attention to certain movements, areas, and motions. Your hands should frame your moves, not detract from them. Be aware of rude gestures in different cultures. Hands can talk!

Footwork

Foot action and foot position can also be used to complete a move. Your feet are the base of your body. They support your body and are vital for movement and posture. Simple movements can be powerful. For example, rocking your weight to one side frees your other leg to move or can allow for easier weight transfer in certain movements. This can make the next step in your routine easier.

The direction your feet point can also say a lot from an audience's perspective. Your feet finish the line of your leg. In some cases, they may complete a line from your arm and down your body too. This makes footwork an aesthetically important consideration.

If done purposefully throughout your act, flexed toes can create a highly skilled performance. Pointed toes can do the same, beautifully finishing the lines you've created. On the other hand, something in between may detract from the shapes your body makes. Cultural difference may influence which foot position is seen as appealing. The same is true for hands. Think of Bollywood, where dainty arms are held out to the side with sharp bends at the wrists. Different cultures have different styles.

Each step and each movement should be purposeful. Don't mess around with extra things. Preserve your energy for the whole routine, and take note of each movement you make.

Body Language

Body language is up there as one of the best forms of communication. Even with language barriers, people can understand it! In fact, it accounts for 60 to 65 percent of all communication. Your body language provides important insight into your character. For a moment we are going to get gender stereotypical here.[2]

Female Body Language

Some signs of attraction:

- tilting the head to the side; this not only shows soft skin but it is like you are letting your natural scent and pheromones out.
- fidgeting with your fingers
- holding a purse in a particular way
- licking your lips.

All of these things are signs of attraction. Even standing with one hip to the side can be a clear communicator! Let the audience see these moves if attraction is what your character is trying to portray.

Try simple things like playing with your hair or arching your back to draw attention to your legs and bust. Give a coy giggle, or sit down on a chair and slide your foot. These movements show interest. When you look back over shoulder, you create a moment. To a degree, mirror imagery can also be seen as flattery when done right. The way you move your legs says something about how your character is feeling, as does the distance between people, the direction you are facing, and the way you use or play with your jewellery. All these movements help to show interest, and they are cues that get used a lot in the world of burlesque performance. Body language and storytelling are important!

Male Body Language

For men, things are a little different. They show interest by raising their eyebrows and may use a strong stance, showing off muscles. Men tend to not lick their lips like women do, but they sometimes part them when they make eye contact instead.

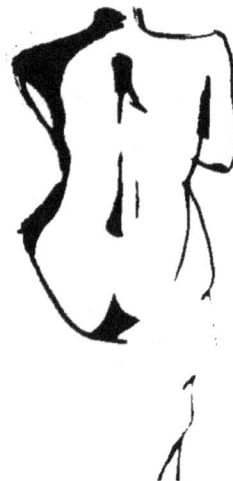

Consider These Cues:

- eye contact
- eyebrow movements
- if you fidget when you sit, you may be seen as uncomfortable, but when you stand it can be portrayed differently.
- smiling or biting your lip
- hand gestures or positions – wriggling can be seen as uncomfortable, whereas fidgeting shows nerves)
- direction of feet, are they pointing at the person or away from them?
- arm placement. Crossed arms is closing your body language, hands on hips is dominant, how do you want to come across?
- body symmetry.

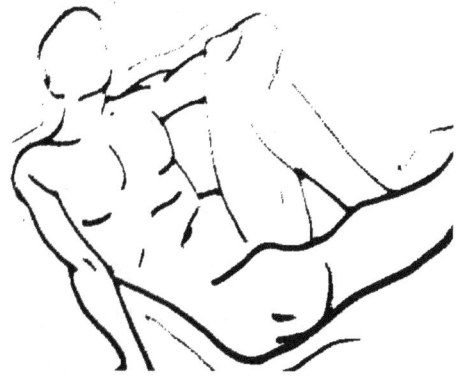

Your whole body speaks, so don't make it look like only half is interested. Open your body to the audience, and show them what is going on in the story. Try to not face your back to the audience, unless on purpose.

My notes:

_____

_____

_____

_____

_____

For Male Performers

- Don't be afraid to be the man on the stage. Don't lose yourself. Embrace it! Give nods to the female performers, but take your spot. This doesn't have to be a show of dominance, but if you are the only male, you don't want to get lost in a sea of dancers. You want to stand out. Embrace the fact that you are different. Be respectful about it, but embody it! Look at the animal kingdom, Male lions and their manes, peacocks and their tails. They are proud and respectful but they stand out in their own right, they don't try and mould in with the crowd.

- If going for sexuality, remember that male sexuality is different from the female experience. Embrace the difference, and don't try to be just another dancer. Just because it is burlesque does not mean that there is a specific way you must move. Just because it is pole doesn't mean you need to move in an exotic way. As much as there are styles of dance, you can make your style stand out from the rest.

- Remember that you will draw attention differently than female dancers do. Once you understand this difference, accept and embrace it. It will help you feel freer in how you move. Males tend to be more visual, whereas females are more about feelings. At the same time, females with an hourglass shape tend to catch a male's eye. This why burlesque places an emphasis on accentuating feminine curves. Females notice muscles instead. Many male performances have a focus on muscles or strength. But this isn't the only way.

- People often try to steer away from stereotypes. Your sexuality is unique, so express it as such. Many women enhance their curves as they saunter onstage. Many men walk onstage showing their muscles. Just because you are male doesn't mean you must show your muscles, and it doesn't mean you have to saunter either. Don't try to be the same as everyone else. Use your attributes, and move in a way that makes you feel good. There will always be critics, but the important thing is to embrace who you are or who your character is.

- Men sometimes feel the need to try harder than women. The truth is that everyone has to work just as hard in dance. Don't let yourself be the novelty guy in the show and coast through. Make a stand with your point of difference.

- Male stereotypes are not challenged enough. This is an opportunity to exaggerate, alter, and explore masculinity. Burlesque is like a safe zone, which is why women have used it to alter femininity. This is now a stereotype itself! What type of stereotype do you want to create for men?

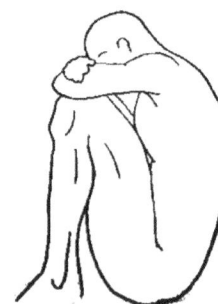

An act is a living, breathing thing. It really is beautiful. Being onstage is a whole other beauty. It is different every performance, even if your routine is structurally the same. The audience is different, and their reactions are different. Your reactions may mirror these differences. It all flows. It's just part of the journey!

Props

- Props are amazing, so don't limit yourself, but remember not to overdo it.
- Going back to burlesque, even a powder puff can be suggestive. Have a love affair with everything, and make the audience want to touch your gloves. Make them think the feather boa is silky. Create tension with your props. Make the audience want to be there too.
- If using props, give them a reason to be there. If you have a pole, why are you going to jump on it? Why is it there? What is its purpose? How does it relate to you? Give your prop a meaning so that it is not just a random item in space that you decided to dance with.
- Make sure you consider the safety aspects of the props you are using. If you need to, consider doing a risk analysis and making any adjustments for the use of your props.
- Using a prop for 5 seconds adds clutter and is often pointless. If you have a prop, use it! Make it have purpose in your routine. It should be there for a reason. Make the most of that, and use it to its full potential.

My notes:

_____

_____

_____

_____

_____

Onstage Thoughts

By the time you're onstage, you should know your act well enough that your thoughts are not just focused on what you're doing unless there is a certain mark you need to hit. This mark may be a musical one, or a literal physical mark on the floor. My mind gets lost in the moment. Sometimes, I know there are key moves coming up, so I will ensure I am facing the camera if I know where the photographer is. Otherwise, I get invested in my act and don't focus on my thoughts.

For **fire performers**, your thoughts should focus on safety and risk management.

- Are there people walking through your space? This is one reason why the fuelling station should always be secure and manned with safe and sealed fuel containers.
- Where are you in your space?
- What is the surface? Are there areas of the ground and your surrounds that pose a risk?
- Is there a high-risk person around you who looks like they might come too close?
- If you hit yourself, are you on fire? Look over to the safety officer now and again to make sure they are paying attention.
- Finally, consider moves and the show. This is why you must rehearse so much ahead of time!

The key is to prepare. If you prepare enough, you can continue when little things go wrong or when something unexpected happens. Prepare enough that the audience doesn't realise there was a mishap. You want to be able to recover and continue, as long as it is safe and appropriate to do so.

Etiquette

- Be charming off the stage and on it. Many deals for work are done backstage. People notice and remember how you treat other cast members and crew. if you had to choose a good performer or a performer who is easy to work with, who would you choose?

- I know it's hard, and I struggle with it too, but try to remember people's names! In character and not in character, the world gets confusing. But remembering names shows respect for your performing community

- People may be excited to see you, but don't let it go to your head. Don't be arrogant about it. People notice!

- Treat the dressing room with respect. There may be many people seeking mirrors or power points to plug in their devices. Others may be trying to use the space, and some may have expensive vintage or heirloom props. People also have allergies, so be respectful when you fill your corner with hairspray. Your venue may have sensitive fire alarms that deodorant could set off, so be mindful of this!

- Keep your stuff compact and together. Taking up half a dressing room is frustrating for other artists. Artists try to keep their stuff together so that they don't lose it and can maintain some form of organisation. This also ensures that no one else touches their belongings. You never know what value a prop or item may have to someone, so don't touch, and keep your stuff together so that people don't feel the need to touch your stuff.

- You'll always need extra hair pins, hairspray, and safety pins in your bag. Hollywood tape can be a saviour too!

- Be aware of what your act involves. Imitation can be flattery, or it can be considered theft! Make your work your own.

- If you are going to do anything unexpected or out of the ordinary, make sure the event and venue staff are aware of it and on your side. There are some rules that shouldn't be pushed, and you need to have respect for these rules. If you are performing something unexpected, there may be extra requirements for the stagehands or someone else. The venue may have expectations as to what they allow. Whether it is a venue, cultural, or safety rule, you need to consider if it is appropriate to break it. Is there risk, and can you manage the risk effectively? Or are you pushing the rules too far? Are you going to promote something that could trigger someone? Or are you referring to a specific group in a negative way? Consider whether this is appropriate.

I did a fire show once where the other performer was using a new prop. She had discussed this with the event organisers and fire safety officers, and they had extra safety staff on board. On top of that, she requested that I join her onstage, doing my own fire routine using the same theme and props but at a lower risk. She explained her act and her concerns, and I agreed. I was like an onstage safety officer. This was a good thing, as halfway through the act, the risk seemed too high. It drew focus to her act and gave it a bit more of a wow factor. I was there to help, so nothing went wrong, as we could communicate about the act and the aspects we were concerned about while onstage. We then extinguished the props we were concerned about before they became an issue. This could only happen because we had event organisers on board and effective risk management processes in place. The safety officers and stagehands were aware of what to expect, and I was onstage to help. Open communication allowed us to perform an unusual routine with highly qualified people around to assist.

Please note that this was a controlled situation with professional insurance and highly experienced performers, as well as multiple trained and experienced fire safety officers and even medical staff present. Do not try experimental things especially if using dangerous substances like fire on your own.

In other instances, I have wanted to have water or bubbles onstage for a dance act, but this was deemed too risky by the venue due to the surface of the floor and the acts that were to follow.

- Be kind and supportive. Performing has many styles, and no style is wrong. If you have a reason to be critical, constructive criticism is amazing when presented correctly. Every person is different, so don't judge others!

- Honour your commitments. Be consistent and polite, and don't quit at the last minute or turn up late. Manage your time. Keep on top of your commitments and availability, and be reliable.

- Be aware of other people's energy. If you need to, create your own little bubble or safe space. Don't let any energy affect you, whether that is someone else's nerves or a backstage diva who expects everyone to do everything for them. Use your safe space to focus on your own energy and keep the vibe high!

- Respect goes a long way. Ensure that you respect everyone's space. They all have their own mental rehearsals and other things going on in their minds. Respect that, and respect everyone else's space.

- Microphone etiquette:
    - At some shows, there are loud noises when someone touches the microphone. The microphone is up to the tech person to control. That is their job, and all the sound will be hooked up through their system. Do not turn the microphone on and off. This will cause it to make loud noises! The tech will turn it on and off for you.
    - Always treat a microphone as live. Assume it is always on. You don't want to get caught with awkward backstage conversations being heard by all.

Act Preparation

- Always know where your show is coming from. You can't be on the road to the future of an art form without knowing its history. You can't do a show about fun when the song is about something sad or angry. Your music choice should match your show. Does the show you are putting together have some history that you need to be aware of while writing it? A well-researched show gains respect.

- Do something different, and challenge yourself. If you get an idea, think about how you can take it further. Break the idea down before putting it together. This will make it stand out more in the end.

- Think about how to stand out. What is your point of difference? Work on that! Stand out from the crowd instead of becoming just another act that will be forgotten after the show.

- We are always learning, so don't stick to what you know. Always try to take it a step further. Learn new skills. Ask for feedback, and take it on board.

- There is no time limit to how long your show must be. It is your show, so prepare and play it the way you feel is most effective.

- Your act doesn't need to start with the music. You can use skills and combinations first. It's up to you. Your performance doesn't have to have a specific style, narrative, or instrumental piece. Choose what you want to portray, the mood it evokes, and the character you are. Consider how these elements relate to you and your relationship to the music.

- It is a visual world, so be creative with your costume, and stand out. If you're a male, there are more options than just a vest and rip-off pants. For girls, think outside the box, especially in the world of burlesque, where the natural expectation has become a corset and a boa. Try not to use too much glitter. Know when your props are too much or when you need to put them in separate acts. Don't overload one show with everything. Create contrast in your costume. Black is flattering, but have something that stands out too. I find it's best to get good-quality clothes. It shows onstage! Remember that lighting can go through things and show what is underneath, especially when clothes are of inferior quality.

- Some colours stand out, while others clash. When looking at your visuals, consider the colours you choose and if they relate to what you are trying to portray. You can play with a colour wheel to see what colours complement or get lost in each other. Remember that opposites attract on the colour wheel! Colours and costumes shouldn't be too busy. You don't want them to get lost in the background or be too confusing. Less is more, and simple stands out!

- Try not to be obvious with your music. A show that uses many of the same old songs is boring. Try to stand out, and make sure you know your music well. Choose timeless music to create a lasting impact with your routine. You want your audience to stay engaged. Remember, you will listen to this song again and again while rehearsing, so make sure you like the song! From when you start putting together your routine, if you hear that song, you will naturally associate it with your act. This goes for your family too. My sister-in-law grew up doing many dance concerts. My husband always along for the ride, now has songs that he has heard so many times that he doesn't want to hear them again.

- If you want to see how music can tell a story, watch Walt Disney's *Fantasia*, a movie that focuses on music, feelings, and the movement of sounds. You can notice the arc of the music. Seeing this relationship can help you visualise how this works. Songs create anticipation in dance. They create dramatic excitement and fill the space.

- Make your show something you would want to see. Would you pay to see your show? How much? Or should you make some adjustments to improve the quality of your performance?

- Remember that many styles of dance are now female-orientated, but men and non-binary people are welcome! Let's make dance, no matter the genre, open and inviting and ensure that everyone is respectful.

- Create elaborate expressions to suit your act and character. Don't do a cutesy face in a non-cutesy act. Your face is part of the act.

- Look at what you're going to do. The audience will look where you look. But don't forget to look at your audience to maintain their involvement. This is a massive part of stage presence.

- Do you want certain photo moments? That is up to you, but you can choreograph certain poses or positions and plan a timed hold for dramatic effect. This can allow for a photo by event photographers.

- If you want to get technical with neatening up your movements, look at planes of movement. This is something to consider when reviewing your routine to ensure that you are using the correct planes. Depending on your act, it can be a focus earlier on.

- People remember the story, the mood, and the feeling of your show. They may not remember the specific moves you used. You want them to remember your confidence in tricks. This is why it is so important to know what your story is and to understand your characterisation. In the end, these elements make a memorable performance. You don't want them talking about how they thought you were going to fall or hurt yourself, you want them amazed by your skill. You want to draw people in, and telling a story or a concept that the audience can relate to or understand, does this. It creates a memorable show amongst all the others.

- Every movement should be with intention. If you are lifting your arm, don't let it just flop in the air as that is where it needs to go. Move it with purpose and emotion, you can even have your own little story or reason as to why it goes there so that every movement is intentional. No matter how small. Intention can make a small movement feel bigger, make it stand out and give it reason.

- Costumes can get smelly from constantly rehearsing in them. Generally, costumes are hand wash only but, on the occasion, where you are wanting just a quick deodorise you can make a spray mix of vodka and water to help reduce that smell. Initially when you spray you will smell the spray, so do this in a well-ventilated area and just lightly mist your costume. You do not need to soak it. I recommend testing this first to ensure there is no reaction to you, or your costume.

- If you use heated creams for muscle tension, just be aware that some of these can remove nail polish. Plan this timing into your preparation, as it is incredibly frustrating to have perfect nails ruined before the show!

- Your heart will feel like it is racing on stage. Slow your moves down, if you do it at what feels normal speed for you, the audience will feel like your show is on fast-forward. As their heartrate is much lower than yours. Take your time.

- Try not to put your trickiest moves in the show if they take all of your energy and concentration. As someone who doesn't perform often, you want to aim for moves that use up to 60% of your ability. This allows room for error and safely correcting the errors without anyone noticing and stuffing everything up. Experienced performers can do moves more up to the 80% of their ability; as they are more experienced at self-correction and the little differences to catch something that may go wrong sooner. Going to 100% means you have less energy to spread across the rest of the routine, you get tired sooner, and have allowed no room for error.

My notes:

_____

_____

_____

_____

_____

_____

High-Risk Performance Preparation

When preparing for an event like a fire show, there is so much to consider, from the ground type to the fabric of curtains and even your costume. You'll need to think about the height of the ceiling, the fuel you're using, and where your fuelling station is. The station must be secure with someone looking after it, and fuel should be sealed/locked at all times.

Plan ahead of time so that you know where your fire safety officer will be and where to find your emergency equipment. Do you know where the venue's emergency equipment is, and are you familiar with emergency procedures? What about the location of a damp cotton towel to extinguish your props? Your fuel spill clean-up kit should be free from the risk of being contaminated and must be clearly labelled. This should be separate from what you use to extinguish flames. Imagine trying to put out a fire in an emergency with an item soaked in fuel! There is a lot to consider when preparing for fire events. This is important not just for you and the venue but also for the audience and the safety officers working with you.

You must consider how many props you need to have prepared and the order in which they will be used. You must ensure that they aren't lit too soon, or you may run out of fuel. How long will your props burn for? Is there an audience exclusion zone? Have you done a hair and costume check? These are all things that come with experience and training, and are some of the reasons why it is so important to get professional training, and professional, experienced high-risk performers- if that is what you are after for your event.

If you are a high-risk performer, there are many pre-show considerations that should not be taken lightly. Insurance is a must, and safety procedures for your own show and venue-specific requirements should always be followed. Every show is different, and so is every venue. Complete a risk analysis for each individual event, working on a case-by-case basis.

Photo by Deric Martin Photography

This is a high-risk performance. In a highly controlled and risk managed environment. Please don't try this at home!

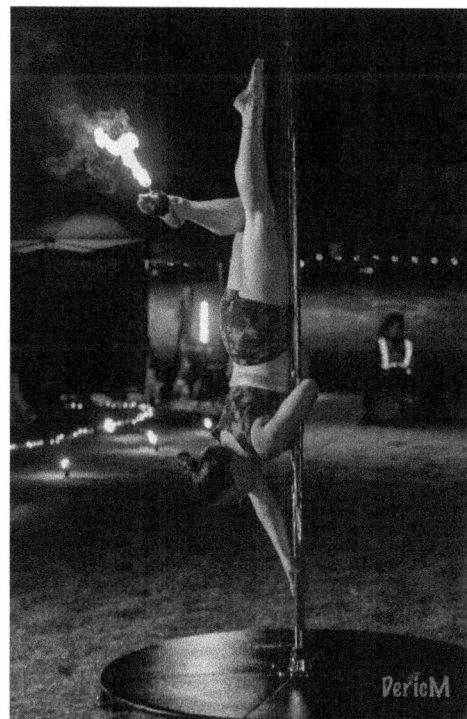

Marketing Your Performance

If marketing is too much for you and you know it isn't your thing, most productions will do marketing for you. However, this is also something you can outsource and get someone else to do on your behalf.

It is all well and good putting on a show, but you need to tell people it's happening in order to have an audience. Some productions will encourage you to invite friends and family to celebrate your performance with you. This is their way of encouraging you to not only create your own support network but also to promote the show and bring people to watch! The more people you get talking about the show, the more people are likely to come along. It's all about networking. This can be done on social media and in person. Some productions even offer incentives for performers and crew to help promote the show. You might get discounted tickets for family members or something else. Be creative with the ways you get people talking. You can try walking adverts or radio and newspaper promotions. You can even advertise on community boards. Contests are another great way to promote your show.

Posters are a helpful way to advertise around town. Use a simple yet eye-catching poster that provides all the relevant details. If the show has a theme or brand, make it stand out so that everyone knows what it is for at first glance. Consistent branding is essential for any performance. Remember that you want to stand out, but you don't want to be overcomplicated. Simplicity is key!

On social media, you still need consistent branding, but you also need to be mindful about when you post. If you start posting too early before details are set, people will forget or get frustrated and lose interest while waiting for more information. You want to build interest in your event so that each time you post about it, the mystery slowly unfolds or the event gets more hype. Demo reels or videos are really good on social media. Ensure you have all information relating to time, cost, cast, venue, and so on. You can use hashtags, venue tags, and location features for your post. Don't fill the page with hashtags. Just ensure you have the key ones there. This method of promoting your show demonstrates that you are serious. As promotion continues, people will get more interested and will start to book tickets.

You want to post things on social media that the audience can engage in. Some posts can be informational, but you should also create engaging posts that invite people to respond to questions. With this type of content, you will get more interaction, and people will look at your post for longer. You can even consider working with social media influencers or brands. In both instances, you want to find a way to add value for everyone.

Want to go old school with signs? That's also an option! Chat to local business owners, homeowners, or even the local government to see if a poster or temporary sign can go up on a busy intersection. You can create street teams to distribute flyers. Ensure they match your brand or stand out in a positive way. Street teams must make a positive impression, whether people are offering flyers or incentives. They must not come across as unprofessional or forceful.

Stickers are fun but can be messy. You want to ensure you aren't the reason for property getting damaged! Magnets are a cool way to promote, as they are easy to remove, and people can take them home to display on the fridge.

Remember to define your audience. Who you are promoting to will depend on how and where you promote. Ensure that you always promote what the show is. You don't want to promote the show as being something it isn't, as this almost guarantees bad reviews! However, if your show or a performer was in a particular event or did something else big, use it! Try words like "as seen in" or "from the artist that brought you ..."

Don't flood your messaging. If you have many things to include, only list three of the main features. You can do another promotion to list others. Too much information can cause key information to get lost. Keep it simple and consistent. There is no reason why you can't use a range of social media platforms, even YouTube, to spread the word about your show!

Consider:

- radio or newspaper advertising
- social media posts, including performer announcements
- PR company support
- advertising through events on social media
- show listings on event websites
- newsletters or mailing lists
- competitions and incentive promotions
- reels or teaser videos on social media
- posters, magnets, and other print promotion
- networking during show intervals and post-show gatherings.

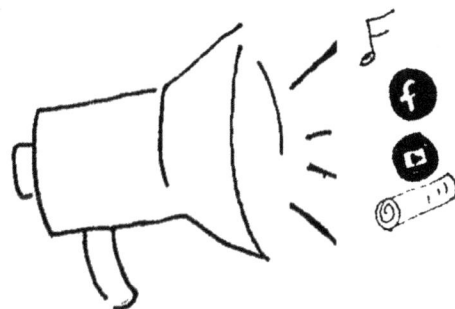

Environmentally Conscious Decisions

Consider your act. Are there ways that you can be more environmentally conscious? Look at creating reusable props instead of single-use items in case you do the show again. Use recycled paper for any paperwork, or use technology instead. You can also get environmentally friendly glitter. Op shops are amazing for costumes, and there are also gifting and sharing groups around the world that may be able to assist with props. Before going out and purchasing something new, consider whether there is a more sustainable way of going about it.

My notes and ideas:

(It is a good idea to note down environmentally friendly suppliers or places you find, so that you remember for next time)

_____

_____

_____

_____

_____

_____

_____

_____

Finance considerations

Budgeting as a creative can be the worst job, but you don't need all the bells and whistles. Making the most of what you have forces you to break down what is important in your show. The most spectacular show doesn't have to have all the flashy elements. It could be black and white and beautifully minimalistic. Remember that less is more. You could be retro and source from an op shop or community groups. Don't think you need all the shiny things! If you have friends and family with skills who can help you create props and costumes, that's great. But don't rely on the same people for help in every show. What is it that your show really needs to work? Does all the fluff add to your story, or does it detract from it? Most of the time, you will find that your show is better with less.

In need of some extra cash to put your show together? You can fundraise! Host quiz nights with other creatives in a similar boat, and split the cost. Talk to local businesses about putting together a raffle, a sausage sizzle, or a movie night. Even consider crowdfunding! Get imaginative, and get yourself organised early enough that these things can happen before there is a last-minute panic. Make a list of clear and achievable goals. How much do you need and for what? Be realistic, and set timeframes and expectations so that you know you are on track to achieve your goals. You should know how much you need, for what, and by when.

Common show production costs are associated with:

- venue hire
- production costs
- equipment
- costumes
- set building
- marketing.

We don't have to stress about that, we aren't producing the show, but it is helpful to know what producers are considering. You are here to create an act. You don't want to expect things from anyone. You want to work out what works best for you. If you do have help, express how grateful you are. But remember not to expect someone else to do all the heavy lifting of setting up props or looking after your set. They are your props, and should be your responsibility. What makes or breaks a show is whether people turn up to see it. Marketing is a huge factor, so support yourself by telling people about your show. Help the show succeed!

The process of word-of-mouth promotion is a great way of networking with other people, performers, and businesses. Consider networking when you think about how you can fundraise, promote, or even source items for your show.

Things to Consider When Looking at Expenses

Are you putting on a show or performing in a show? As a performer, your expenses are very different from those of a producer, but it's good to have a vague idea of how much goes on behind the scenes. This gives you respect for the organisers. In relation to performing, the costs are variable. You can plan and budget how much you feel is appropriate to spend. As an event organiser, you will need to juggle a range of fixed and variable costs.

As a Performer, You'll Need to Consider:

- hair, nails, and makeup costs
- costume and accessory costs
- cost of props or specialty equipment
- cost of fuel and parking at the event or rehearsals
- training space (if relevant)
- performer insurance.

As an Event Organiser, Additional Considerations Include:

- music licence
- liquor licence
- insurance for the event
- photographer and videographer
- lighting, sound, and other technology and technicians.
- Riggers, if aerial acts are being performed
- stage manager, MC, and stagehands
- security and ticket staff
- venue hire for event and rehearsals. Venue considerations include: space, size, flooring and capacity standing/seating and what equipment the venue supplies etc.
- seating availability
- advertising and marketing (including graphic designers, photographers, artists etc)
- other registration fees or taxes.

It's important not to undercut the industry with your fee. People will pay for a quality show, and if you undercut the industry standards, people start having to work for less, or businesses accept lower-quality performers. In some industries, especially if you are a fire or high-risk performer, this could also be a safety risk, as performing experience and safety aspects may not be understood or prepared for.

I perform one volunteer show per year for a cause close to my heart, and I explain this to people when they ask me to perform. This is not a pre-determined cause, but it is something I judge as opportunities arise. This seems to be quite well respected and understood. We have an industry of our own, and we respect our industry. It is work, and it takes a lot of time, effort, and training. Performers should be paid appropriately for their work. Undercutting the industry by charging less than you should doesn't just affect everyone else; it also ends up affecting you.

Don't be afraid to say no! Know your boundaries, and stick to them. Understand the reasons behind your boundaries so that you can explain them if you need to. Ensure all negotiations are clear, and write everything down. A clear contract ensures that you know where you stand and what you have agreed to. It also means that producers and organisers know their obligations. As you evolve and grow, things change, so be aware that your boundaries may shift too. Always be clear about your expectations and requirements. Performing is business, and time is money. Businesses need to know what they're paying for, and you need to know where you stand. It may be a fun business to be in, but that doesn't mean you can relax on boundaries.

Your Health

The leadup to a show can be stressful. Ensure you prioritise your health and well-being, getting a good amount of sleep and eating a healthy, balanced diet. Also consider your mental health. If you need to step away and have a break, do it. You may find you come back feeling refreshed and inspired. Don't run yourself into the ground so that you are at risk of getting ill before the show. Ensure you have time to recharge. If you need to sit and gather your thoughts and mentally prepare yourself before the show, do it. You have set your goals and managed your expectations.

Remember to balance your training and rehearsing to not tire out and fatigue your body, if your muscles need a warm bath to recover, then don't put that off. Also consider longevity of your muscles and joints, balance your stretching with conditioning. Ensure you do your prehab exercises to keep your joints and body safer for longer, don't wait until you have an injury strengthen and maintain your body first.

Performing is a business, and there are occupational health and safety considerations to keep in mind, as well as risk management for your performances. Ensure that you keep yourself, your audience, and fellow performers and stagehands safe. Understanding and managing risks is key to a safe performance. As long as you are physically safe and mentally prepared, you can take the next step. Now it's time to perform!

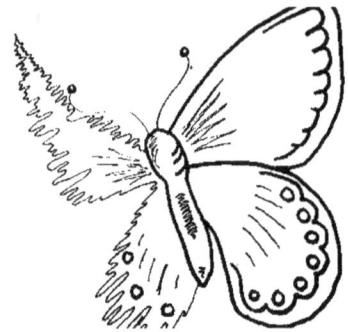

Create a Training Schedule

Work out how long you have until your performance and how long you have to finalise your routine. Know when you need to start practising with props, and break this all down so that you know how many days a week and for how long you need to schedule training sessions. Even if a practice session is not physical, make time to work on music, visuals, costumes, and prop creation. Even put time aside to make notes from watching your video recordings. Every day, take one more step towards your goal, leaving plenty of time to spare.

You can schedule your time in a range of ways. You can set a day for off-the-pole training and a session for floorwork. I tend to block sections together so I have a combination I work on regularly to get it all in my muscle memory. Then I pair that with a spin combination or a lower-impact combination. This means that I don't overwork my body. Once the more advanced stuff starts to come more easily, I change up what I train and rehearse sections of the routine together. I find I need to get the intricate combinations sorted first to be able to do this. Otherwise, I am constantly thinking about what comes next.

Remember to only use moves you can achieve. Allow room for error. Even the best performers often only perform to 80 percent of their ability, as things could change on the night, and you don't want to be stretched to your limit.

Remember to allow rest days. You don't want to make your body too tired to perform and risk injuries. Look after your body, and make sure you sleep and eat well! Sleep helps your body repair and regenerate from all the physical training you do. If your sleep decreases, your risk of injury increases. It isn't just about your physical health. It's about mental health too!

Training is about quality, not quantity. Any high-intensity training should be followed by rest. If you need to train the following day after a high-intensity session, either make it low intensity or use a different style of movement to rest areas of your body. If there is a skill you want to hammer away at, look at what other cross-training exercises you can do to assist. Could yoga or Pilates help? What about resistance-band training? Look for ways to vary your training instead of constantly drilling the same moves and fatiguing your muscles. You need to ensure diversity of movement and avoid overworking your body.

Please keep in mind the age of younger performers when organising training plans. The younger the dancer, the more rest time their body will need. This is due to them not having the life experience to know when to stop and rest yet. This needs to be taught to them. Studies have shown that youth between 8-16 years should only train a maximum hours per week to match their age. Meaning a 10-year-old, should train 10 hours per week maximum. Otherwise risk a 70% increased chance of injury. [1]

Stage one of training for a show is the hard bit. This is when you actually get up and get to the studio to train. Once you are at the studio, stage two begins when you work out what you are going to work on. Where is your mind and your body at that day? Not everyone works well with structured plans. The important thing is to constantly make progress, a little bit at a time. Knowing why you want to perform and why you are there is a good driving force to help you channel creative energy. It also helps if there are others involved to encourage you. Some performers may be motivated by the experience. Others may be driven by networking or want to build a reputation or trial a new concept. Knowing what drives you really helps you stay on track.

Sometimes things never feel done, but you need to set yourself limits, deadlines and allow yourself to "finish" each section, or the routine. Then you can practice, work on lines, neatening it up and you will end up with a finished looking product. But that takes time, so put some limitations on when your choreography is finished, so you have the time to neaten and add the extra flourishes to the moves.

POLE
WORKOUT
PLANNER

RAPTURE
Arts

POLE GOAL

MONDAY	TUESDAY	WEDNESDAY

THURSDAY	FRIDAY	SATURDAY

Rapture Arts

Mental Preparation

Positive self-talk in the lead-up to a show is important. Accept the nerves, and envision a fantastic performance. Plan to deal with unexpected surprises positively. No one else knows your routine, so no one knows when you mess up. You can keep going and flow on. In a competition, perform like you have already won. The audience will notice when you are unsure, so go in with confidence. Relax, think positively, and train until the moves are in your muscle memory so that you can have fun onstage. If you want to, you can visualise the audience's reaction once the routine is done to prepare for the show.

Know your routine, and have your props and costume ready. Plan when to get to the venue, and know what you need. Make sure all your paperwork is done ahead of time. Knowing that you have this sorted will make things feel a lot easier to manage.

Do you have anything you feel you may need to do to help mentally prepare? Note them down here so that you remember.

_____

_____

_____

_____

_____

_____

_____

_____

_____

_____

_____

Use Video to Neaten Up

Videos are the only way you can see your routine in the leadup to your show. This helps you clean up your act and remove fluff. It also helps you see if your props are working effectively or if there are any costume adjustments needed. You can use videos to pick up flexed toes, hand positions, bent knees, or lines in your body that aren't quite right. You can even use video to analyse body position and the position of the audience. This can help you perfect transition changes and make flow adjustments. This is how little elements are pulled apart and put back together. Videos will never be the same as a performance, but this is the closest you can get to seeing yourself, allowing you to create the performance you are imagining.

I suggest making notes, as the more you see yourself, the less you will notice the little things. First impressions are important, so make note of the things you want to fix. Fix them, re-record your routine, and evaluate it again. Don't do this to the point where it is no longer fun. Honestly, I rarely video my routines, but it is so helpful to be able to see what you look like from an external perspective. Video is a fantastic tool to help you neaten up your routine.

You can even look at videoing sections of your routine. This way, you can put everything into each section and perform to the best of your ability without fatigue. Your fitness and stamina will increase as you train and practise. By viewing each section at its best, you'll get a more accurate picture of what you're aiming to achieve. If you have a video editor, you can edit video to put sections together. This way, you can watch all sections together and see how the flow works. Isolating sections also helps you focus on one part and perfect it before moving on to the next.

Final Checks

Once you have your choreography and musicality, you're almost ready to finalise your routine. There are a few things you should keep an eye on with regard to technique.

- Are your toes pointed or flexed?

- How are your lines and angles? Are your legs straight? Do you have long lines across your body, or are you happy with the angles in the routine?

- What about hand placement? Do you have a wandering hand, or does it have a purpose?

- When you bring your arm around, does it follow a nice flow, or can you make this more purposeful?

- What about your facial expression? Can you relax and breathe, or are you in character? Can you portray emotion in your expression and performance?

- Are you happy with how you have used your space? Do you have an entry and exit plan? Are you using the whole space? Or are you saturating one area? Using the stage, and they way you use the stage helps to set the energy for the show. Moments of still should be purposeful, even full of dramatic effect.

- Is there any fluff? Or does every move contribute to the overall flow and structure of your routine? You only have a few minutes on stage, so you want every step, every gesture to be worth it.

- How are your transitions? Are they smooth and purposeful? Harnessing transitions is so important. They are part of your act! Transitions can be the thing to make or break the act.

- Rehearse as if you're performing. This helps you prepare for the show. Prepare to create an experience onstage, looking for connection and emotional response. These things won't show up in your video, on stage you can extend moments, emphasise certain movements or points in the music so much easier than on video. As well as actually being able to connect with the audience, these are things we need to visualise and mentally prepare for.

- Visualise and prepare yourself. What will a successful show look like to you? How will it feel?

- Remember, only you know your act. If you mess up, flow with it. Maintain character and professionalism, and keep going. No one else will know, so don't make it obvious!

You may find that checklists help to ensure that you have covered all elements of dance technique and themes within your routine. Feel free to make your own, listing what you want to achieve so that you can reflect on your routine and ensure you have achieved what you set out to. Here is an example of what you can include on a checklist.

Act Creation by Lara Johnson

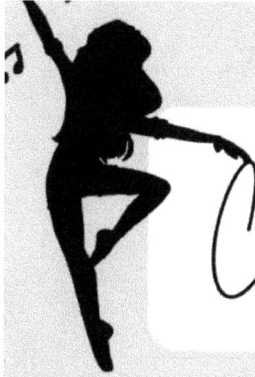

Choreography Checklist

- [ ] Use of dynamic levels (floor, air, standing, etc.)
- [ ] Range of elements used (time, space, energy etc.)
- [ ] Use of varied body shapes and lines
- [ ] Beginning and ending pose matches theme and style
- [ ] Unexpected or interesting movements choreographed in
- [ ] Use of planes of movement (vertical horizontal and sagittal)
- [ ] Choreography communicates idea and theme
- [ ] Choreography matches music, and is chosen to not offend
- [ ] Contains elements of movement, travelling , static, uses pauses effectively
- [ ] Effective use of stage, as well as audience acknowledgement
- [ ] Focus points, or wow moments included (again pauses here)
- [ ] Practiced with costuming &props ensuring flow and ease
- [ ] Well rehearsed so that the steps are more natural meaning that the personality can come out on stage

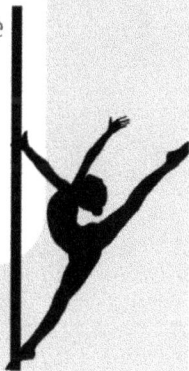

#RaptureArts

Act Creation by Lara Johnson

Feel Free to write your own Checklist here:

☐ _____
☐ _____
☐ _____
☐ _____
☐ _____
☐ _____
☐ _____
☐ _____
☐ _____
☐ _____
☐ _____
☐ _____

Providing Information

When you're signing up to work on a show, there are some general details required. This is after liability waivers, and you will already have all information you need for the show. Information is required so that the people putting the show together know how to balance it. This may influence who performs when or help accommodate the time needed to set up and pack up. Details may also provide staff with time to get music and lights in order. Information may help the MC and stagehands, providing them with a clear sense of what they need to say or do to help the show run smoothly.

It helps to have an idea of what will be asked of you so that it doesn't feel overwhelming or strange. It's just part of putting your act in a show. It's important not to hand information in at the last minute, as marketing staff may need it to advertise the show. There are many people involved behind the scenes, and they very much appreciate being able to do their jobs without a last-minute panic. Imagine if every performer handed in their sheet at the last minute. It would be utter chaos! Not just the stage managers, but the lighting, sound, marketing, all sorts of people would be affected by last minute changes or getting information late. Remember, you don't have to do anything you aren't comfortable with. If you are asked to, stand your ground, and do not allow yourself to compromise your personal boundaries.

Being aware of these considerations and preparing for them gives you a professional appearance. It means that event organisers don't have to go back and forth to get information, making you easier to work with.

It is also worth re checking the event details... Are there any particular criteria that you need to meet for your event? Or event specific details that you need to note?

Performer Contact Details		
Real name(s):		
Daytime phone(s):	Mobile phone(s):	
Email address:		
Act Details:		
Stage name(s):		
Comp's full name (you get one free ticket):		
Name of your act (optional):		
Any special way you (or your group) would like to be announced, other than by your stage name?		
Gender pronouns: (his/him/he, her/she, they/them etc)		
Describe your act:		
Act Requirements:		
Will you be using large props? Do you need anything set up onstage before you start your act, or do you have any special requirements for your act?		
Will you be leaving props or costume items on the stage when you finish your act?		
Is assistance required during your act?		

Music:		
Length of the song:	Song name:	Artist:
When do you want your music to start?	When you are onstage? When you are offstage?	Do you want music to fade out/stop before track finishes? If so, when (timestamp)?
Describe if necessary:		
How/In what format will you be supplying your music?		
Is there a lighting cue?		
What is the music timestamp for any lighting changes?		
Other Act Specifics:		
What colour is your costume(s)?		
Is there anything else we should know?		
Are you starting onstage or offstage?		

Act Creation by Lara Johnson

Your Performance Emergency Pack

- Baby wipes and deodorant are optional if you get nervous sweats and need to freshen up.

- Depending on costuming, I sometimes carry a hot glue gun for last-minute repairs. I also bring superglue for shoe malfunctions, stored in a Ziploc bag so it doesn't risk damaging anything if it breaks. I recommend inspecting props and costumes before leaving for the venue, however accidents happen and I have seen these items used enough back stage to always have them with me.

- Bring a hair brush and makeup, including:
    - nail glue
    - eyelash glue
    - hair pins
    - safety pins
    - a small mirror
    - makeup removal pads.

- Pack your own snacks. Be aware of common allergens and food that makes a mess.

- Carry a drink bottle. Many venues don't have access to drinking water backstage, so have some of your own, just in case. This also means that you can pick a bottle that doesn't smudge your makeup!

- Bring a dressing gown or large jacket to put over your clothes. This is a big help if you need to run back to the car. But also to keep you warm backstage after you have done your warm up.

- Always carry an emergency sanitary item.

- It's also a good idea to bring an electrolyte tablet, especially if you're performing in the heat!

My notes:

_____

_____

_____

_____

_____

Act Creation by Lara Johnson

Show Day Preparation

Olympic athletes train, prepare, and focus. But one aspect you don't often think about is visualisation! You get there, and you know what you're going to do, but the crowd and the atmosphere are next level. Did you prepare for that? Did you visualise how it would feel to walk out and have everyone watching and cheering, the air buzzing with anticipation? No matter how well you know your art, this can make the world of difference. Mental preparation is a big deal. So how can you prepare for show day?

First, rehearse. Know what you are doing inside out. Once you know it and show day is in sight, treat every rehearsal day like a show day so it isn't a shock. Replicating that day in the weeks leading up to it helps you prepare mentally and reduce nerves. Part of this mental and physical preparation includes getting to know your props. If you have a specific prop, train with it so that you get used to its weight, size, grip and so on. This is also true for hair styles and costumes, even a certain hair clip can feel odd or get in the way if you haven't trained with it on prior to the performance. It's fine to train with a dump prop initially while waiting for your prop to arrive or be finalised, but in the end, you must practise with what you will use onstage.

Work out when you perform best. After a few days off? Or a few days into training? When do you feel best on your training days? Design your show prep to suit your routine, keeping in mind the need for tech runs. Keeping a record of your training and scheduling rest days will help you feel more confident with what you are doing. Notice patterns, and make adjustments to reduce the fear of a bad day on show day. Also take note of how much stretching or what dynamic movements you can easily do back stage to keep warm whilst waiting for your time to go on stage.

When show day arrives, don't change anything. You have been preparing for this! Warm up, and stretch. Replicate your routine from training. Ensure that you cover every muscle group you need for the show, keeping everything balanced. Do you have a certain time when you put grip aid on before training? Make sure you take note of this so that you can replicate it prior to the show.

Eating is a big thing, and it can totally damage your lipstick—and your breath. Then there is the issue of bloating, or the worry of having something stuck between your teeth. For this reason, I love trail mixes and fruit. Eat something that provides energy but is light and won't make you feel heavy, full, or bloated. You want a snack before the show, but nerves generally mean you won't want much more. Make sure you eat afterwards, and don't get lost in the buzz of performing. Generally, it's best to have a snack 30 or 40 minutes before the show, but this will vary depending on your body. Make it a habit to also do this in your rehearsals so that you know what time is right for you.

Allow time! You don't want to be stressed or rushed. Plan time for hair, makeup, and costuming. Work out where you are getting ready. Brush your teeth before you leave the house. Will you get dressed at home or at the venue? What do you need to bring? Do you need power? Will you have access to power? Do you need to bring a power board so that you can share a power point? Do you have an emergency pack of hair pins, safety pins, double-sided tape, and anything else you'll need? Plan to be ready well in advance so you can warm up and get in the zone. Don't forget to allow time for an emergency toilet run before the show!

Once you are warmed up and ready, keep an eye on your run sheet. Know when you need to be onstage. Remember, you still need to keep yourself warm! I like to wear a big cloak or a dressing gown backstage, but a tracksuit is also awesome if you don't wear shoes. Choose something with a zip, as you don't want to pull anything over your head and mess up your hair. Ensure that whatever you wear to keep warm won't compress or damage your costume.

You can do some light jogging or other workouts while you wait. For pole, you will already know how your skin grips best and how to get to that point of warmth and maintain it. You'll know what level of tack you need for your skin to grip effectively. Try to maintain that. Make sure your hands aren't so dry that you slip, and make sure they aren't sweaty and slippery. Maintain whatever level of dewiness is right for your skin to have its optimum grip.

Breathe! Relax! Enjoy it! You're here because it is fun, not because it is a chore. You want to be here. You have prepared physically and mentally. You've got this!! Take a few breaths, close your eyes, and get yourself into your character. The second you step onstage, that is who you are, and it is all about you! Be the character, soak it up, and remember to have fun!

Make sure you thank the stagehands and anyone who has helped you at the side of the stage. A little gratitude goes a long way! If you act like a diva, it gets noticed. Working behind the scenes is a stressful job, so help where you can, and say thank you to those who help you.

My notes:

_____
_____
_____
_____
_____
_____
_____
_____
_____
_____
_____
_____
_____
_____
_____
_____

Pre-Show Jitters

Feeling nervous? This is totally normal! There are a few things you can do to help.

- Look over the top of the audience instead of looking at the people watching.

- Have you read Harry Potter? Imagine the charm for boggarts. This makes scary things look funny instead! (It follows the same principle that you hear in movies, of imagining the audience naked.) If you need to look at them, you want it to not feel overwhelming and scary.

- Focus on your mission and the onstage world you create. Push all other thoughts out of your mind.

- Practise until you know your routine and the music well so that you aren't stressed about what comes next.

- Have fun. If you enjoy your performance, the audience will too. Your vibe is contagious!

- Stop internalising your thoughts, and focus on external factors. Get back into the rhythm of the song. Find fluidity in the movement.

- Visualisation is the key. Visualise everything going smoothly and feeling effortless. Use training to prepare for show conditions. Like turning a little mental switch to make your rehearsals important, even film for showreels to increase the importance of the rehearsal. This can make the real show feel less stressful.

- One thing you can do for nerves before you step on stage; is to trick your body into creating a calming response. Think about when you are crying and you tend to take a second breath in as you are calming after. We can do this same thing to help calm us from our nerves. Take a big breath in, then when your lungs are full of air, try and take another short breath in. Then breathe out. Can you feel the tension ease? It doesn't work for everyone, but is a tool that is used by many.

Pre show rituals are a big thing to assist with nerves. Some people meditate in a corner, some people pace, others like to chat and relax with people. Everyone's pre-show experiences are different and we need to respect that. Do you need a moment of quiet before walking on stage, or are you shaking all your jitters out and jumping the energy around before taking a breath and walking purposely on stage? Working out what works for you will help create your own little pre-show routine and make things feel more manageable.

As the curtains draw back, light streams onto the stage. The air is buzzing, and the audience is cheering. It feels electric. You look out at the shadows in the audience. You pause for a moment as the prickles of your goosebumps match the electricity in the air. You realise that you can't actually see anyone in the audience. Suddenly, the music starts. It's like a switch has been turned on, and the momentary pause has ended. Your act has begun. The character within you appears out of nowhere. The bounce returns to your step and the energy to your face and body as you feel your posture lift. A world of your own creation surrounds you onstage. Invite the audience in, and introduce them to your world. This space is yours!

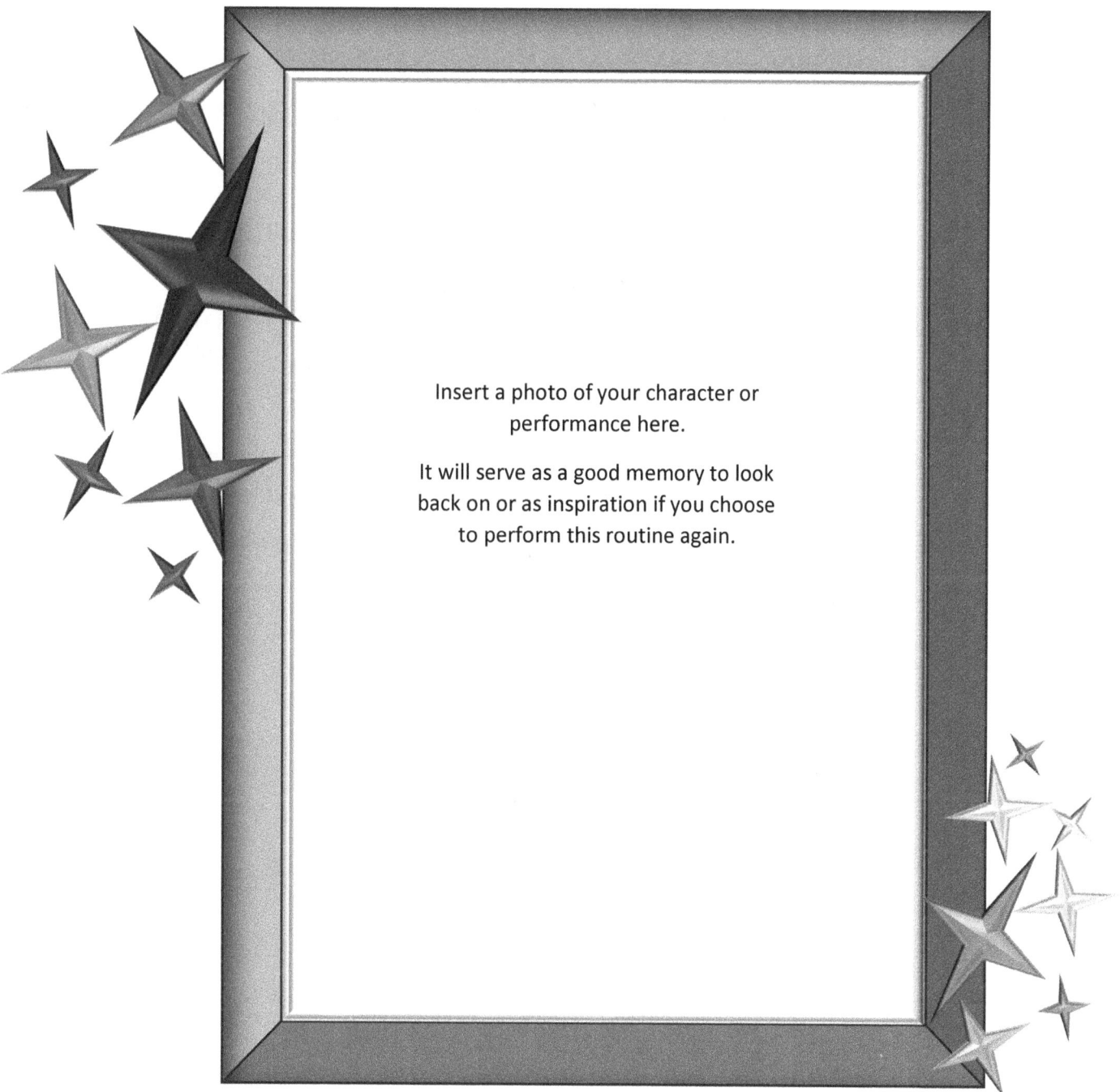

Take a bow, and thank your audience, as well as the sound and lighting crew and any other technicians and helpers. Give a wave of acknowledgement, or applaud in their direction. This show came together because a lot of people worked on it and more came to see it. Thank everyone for being a part of this experience.

You made it!

Insert a photo of your character or performance here.

It will serve as a good memory to look back on or as inspiration if you choose to perform this routine again.

Post-Show Care

This is something that is often forgotten. You spend so long working towards an event that you can feel somewhat lost after it. Set your boundaries, and within those boundaries, celebrate with other performers after the show. Share the buzz and the energy with them. That way, you aren't just heading home to stillness, which may be a bit of a shock. It can sometimes feel like a lonely path, but you have a community of like-minded people around you. They can share your feelings, and you can go through this experience together. Remember that everyone will have an opinion on your act or want to know about it. Don't let it get to you. You did the best you could, and that is the most important thing. Make sure you look after yourself over the next few days. Have a bath, and treat yourself to a celebratory dinner or a small treat. Ease yourself back into everyday life. Appreciate the moments you had onstage. Share the joy, and be grateful for the opportunity.

Not quite sure what is going on or what I am talking about? When you lead up to a performance the world seems extra shiny. So much excitement and anticipation and thus there is little pumps of adrenaline into your system. So, it is natural for things to appear dull, heavy or lethargic after the event. The body needs to re-balance after the extra adrenaline and high energy focus. This lull is a natural response driven by the Parasympathetic Nervous system. Part of coping with it is being aware of it! Whether you have catch up time with performers or go through the photos of the event. You can even plan some rest time, some time for you or shift focus to the next exciting focus. You can plan little check ins with friends or other performers, or even a time to sit and check in with yourself. These all help get through a potential week of post-performance-come-down.

Notes of Reflection:

General:

_____

_____

_____

_____

_____

_____

What I really liked:

_____

_____

_____

_____

_____

_____

What I can improve or adjust:

_____

_____

_____

_____

_____

_____

_____

Networking notes:

Connections made, where they are from and other networking notes:

_____

_____

_____

_____

_____

_____

Anything I need to follow up from the performance:

_____

_____

_____

_____

_____

_____

_____

Reference:

As this is mostly from a lifetime of personal experiences from myself and others, there aren't many scientific journals needed to research and reference. There is however information out there on training schedules, training styles, body and muscle fatigue and care as well as injury prevention. There is also a range of research done on stereotypes and body language if it is something that interests you.

1. *American Medical Society for Sports Medicine – Intense, Specialized Training in Young Athletes Linked to Serious Overuse Injuries - 16-Apr-2013 10:00 AM EDT, by Loyola Medicine*
2. *https://www.psychologytoday.com/au/blog/cutting-edge-leadership/202204/how-men-and-women-flirt-body-language (How Men and Women Flirt with Body Language - April 3, 2022 Ronald E. Riggio Ph.D)*

Act Creation by Lara Johnson

Thank you for taking this journey with me. I hope you have managed to take some key points or techniques and ideas out of this workbook to use in your future performances.

Enjoy the journey, and make the most of the moments you create. To others, they may appear magical, and to be the creator of magic is something special. I feel very privileged to be a stepping stone in your journey. Thank you, and good luck with your future performing endeavours!

Lara
xxx